MW00748923

REQUIEM FOR MY BROTHER

REQUIEM *for* *my* BROTHER

Marian Botsford Fraser

GREYSTONE BOOKS

DOUGLAS & MCINTYRE PUBLISHING GROUP

Vancouver/Toronto/Berkeley

Greystone Books
A division of Douglas & McIntyre Ltd.
2323 Quebec Street, Suite 201
Vancouver, British Columbia
Canada V5T 4S7
www.greystonebooks.com

Library and Archives Canada Cataloguing in Publication
Fraser, Marian Botsford, 1947–
Requiem for my brother / Marian Botsford Fraser.

ISBN-13: 978-1-55365-008-9 · ISBN-10: 1-55365-008-5

1. Botsford, John Davis, 1949–2001. 2. Multiple sclerosis—Patients—
Canada—Biography. 3. Fraser, Marian Botsford, 1947– —Family.   I. Title.
RC377.F63 2006   362.196′8340092   C2006-904576-3

Editing by Nancy Flight
Copyediting by Iva Cheung
Jacket design by Courtenay Webber
Text design by Naomi MacDougall
Jacket photograph by J.H. Botsford
Printed and bound in Canada by Friesens
Printed on acid-free paper that is forest friendly (100% post-consumer
recycled paper) and has been processed chlorine free.
Distributed in the U.S. by Publishers Group West

The following publishers have given permission to use quoted material:
Lines from the song *Helpless* by Neil Young, copyright Neil Young. Reprinted by permission of Wixen Music/Alfred Permissions. Lines from *Beowulf: A New Verse Translation*
by Seamus Heaney. Copyright © 2000 Seamus Heaney. Reprinted
by permission of W.W. Norton & Company.

We gratefully acknowledge the financial support of the Canada Council
for the Arts, the British Columbia Arts Council, and the Government
of Canada through the Book Publishing Industry Development Program
(BPIDP) for our publishing activities.

There is a town in north Ontario
With dream, comfort, memory to spare...
NEIL YOUNG

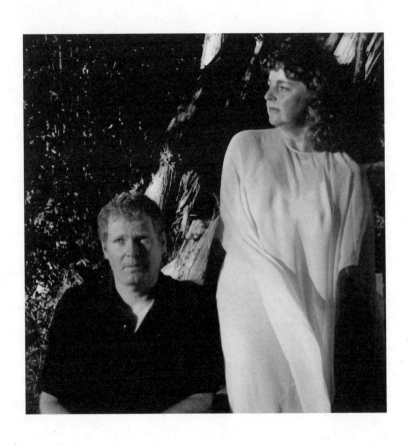

CONTENTS

THIS RAIN, THIS RAIN, THIS RAIN. Ten, eleven hours of it, on the tin roof, dripping off the jack pine and the spruce and the edge of the narrow porch, running in rivulets down the paths and through the bush to the lake. Rolling off the white kayak overturned on the dock, only dimly visible in the mist. Filling the lake, which ripples and riffles in spots but is mostly a sheet of slate, silvery when there is a brief glimmer of light in the sky to the north. For a while the loon is there, but then gone. Shoreline comes and goes as the rain crescendos, diminuendos. Not even a visible cloud, just a gray sheet pulled over the sky.

Rain pours all afternoon, through the calcified memories and the muddy ones. All evening, five candles and three lamps, lit by six in the failing, wet light. Even the hummingbird is daunted by this downpour. The chipmunk is silenced. Long after darkness falls, the loon makes a forlorn comment, only twice. No loon answers.

Long-forgotten thoughts wash up, images packed away in powdery boxes, now loosened by the rain.

Finally, around ten in the evening, the rain stops. There is still the sound of dripping and the smell of thick, moist air and damp bark. Small lapping waves on the little beach. A whiff of wood smoke. And then the rain begins again, a hesitant little trickle, gentle shower escalating into a downpour, a limitless bounty of soft, sluicing water.

What surfaces . . .

BLESS

THIS

HOUSE

DAWN. I awaken suddenly from a deep sleep to thunder—the heavy, waterlogged kind, hard to situate on the lake. It is hot and muggy, oppressive. There is sporadic, needlelike lightning on the horizon and an ash-colored filter on the sky. Is there a tiny breeze, or is that a brief scatter of rain?

I am sleeping on the floor of the screen porch, facing the lake, visible through a light lattice of birch trees. The rest of the family is scattered around the cottage we have rented on Lake Kenogami, not far from the town of Kirkland Lake. My sister, Sara, is in one bedroom; her oldest son, Jon, and his wife, Suki, upstairs in a bedroom; her younger sons, Quinn and Gideon, in sleeping bags on sofas or mattresses; my daughter, Katherine, in the screen porch with me. I am always the first to wake up.

Slip out the door, down the lawn, barefoot and silent to the end of the dock, trying not to disturb the duck that sits there, discard my T-shirt and climb down the little ladder into the lake. A vestigial breath of mist rests on the motionless water. Swim out—breast stroke, no splashing—until I am about 100 meters from shore. Turn my back to the thunder, lie perfectly still, arms sculling lazily, toes pointing skyward, the way our father always got such pleasure out of floating.

It is Monday morning of the long weekend in August, twenty-two days and twelve hours since the death of our brother, Dave. I have never known time to pass so slowly.

Not long for this world . . .

Dave's funny old diver's watch with the ragged Velcroed strap weighs on my wrist. It lay on my kitchen counter in Toronto from the day of his death until this past Friday, when we collected our children from the airport and drove up north. It is indestructible, the watch that has never stopped, never needing a new battery in the twenty years he wore it. It sounds only the hour and half-hour—one beep, two beeps. I have decided, without thinking too deeply, to consign it to the black waters of Lake Beaverhouse with Dave's ashes.

An early riser on a dock two cottages down raises his coffee mug to me in silent salute. I wave, then float, eyes closed, until I hear sounds of my family stirring in the cottage. I know the children are waking with a jumble of emotions about the day ahead. They don't know what to expect, and the weight of their mothers' sorrow silences their usual blunt curiosity. This is a plan Sara and I idly sketched out in my garden in Toronto on a hot July afternoon, without an

2

inkling that Dave would die within hours that same evening. The children have never been where we will go today.

It preys incessantly on my mind that I did not ever discuss this plan with Dave. We never spoke of death.

The shadow-stalker, stealthy and swift...

Day and night I have a shadow who grieves and silently
wails. Hovers in the wings while the daily drama unfolds as
it must. My heart is leaden, but head and body are smoothly
running engines—writing obituaries, transporting ashes,
making notes and lists, calling, packing, and giving his
things away, doing legal things. Renting a van, renting a
cottage, a boat, packing for the trip north, coordinating the
travel of children from three cities, secretly assembling all
the elements for Sara's birthday celebration, driving, singing loudly in the car to obscure the clicking sound of thaw-
ing lobsters, spraying lavender mist to obliterate the scent
of fifty orange and pink and yellow roses inexorably opening. Each second is a heartbeat.

The roses are full-blown now and their scent untram-
meled; they are gathered into loose bouquets on a table on
the deck. It was Sara's fiftieth birthday on Saturday. We hid
everything in the back of the van for the eight-hour drive,
and the day of her birthday we executed a perfect celebration that ended in a supper of lobster and champagne and
small New York cheesecakes smothered in wild blueberries,
made by the owner of the bar on Lake Kenogami. Then we
had presents around the table; her gift from Dave and me
was a 1938 copy of her favorite childhood book, for which
she had been searching for years: *Li'l' Hannibal,* which our

3

mother read to her every morning as she brushed her long red hair into fat, springy ringlets. Sara read it aloud by candlelight in a wobbly voice. We leaned in and listened silently and the darkness wrapped us. It seemed Dave was not really absent, honoring with us her birthday, his death day.

Now it is what we already refer to as "Dave's Day." The sun has burned off the mist and the thunder has subsided. God has stopped moving the furniture around upstairs.

After breakfast, we collect the things we will need: picnic supplies, life jackets, insect repellent and hats and sunscreen and sunglasses, swimsuits, camera, plastic glasses and champagne for a toast. The photo album that Sara assembled in the days after Dave's death and the two little cedar boxes containing his ashes. Last evening at Wayne's cottage down the lake, Sara and I were told of a strict fire ban (I'd seen a sign in the local store, but it had not registered), so Wayne had phoned around to people on the lake and found us a propane stove. "It'll be sitting outside Dave Hurd's garage tomorrow morning, and he's right down at the end of your road." We are all in the van and on the road exactly as we had planned, by 9:45.

Dave Hurd's wife, Linda, is on her tractor mower when we pull into their driveway; she is a stranger with shiny black hair and a round, serene face, not originally from Kirkland Lake. She gives me the little propane stove, a wrench to open the gas canister, and a few brief instructions. I nod politely, scarcely absorbing her words. I stand paralyzed for a moment, so she guides me gently to my side of the car.

4

"I heard your brother rumbling this morning," she says, smiling, "in anticipation of the day."

"I hope it doesn't rain," I say to her as I get into the van.

"It won't rain," she says, as if she knows for sure.

We drive east, straight through Kirkland Lake. The two cedar boxes are in a red embroidered tapestry bag that sits between Sara and me in the front seat. The children doze in the back seats—Jon and Katherine both 25, Suki 30, Gideon almost 19, and Quinn just 14.

For Sara and me the dissonance between the town we grew up in and the current reality is exquisitely painful and registered unwittingly at every turn in the road, every stoplight and boarded-up building and ghostly landmark. When we were young, this town was a busy, proud place; there was a community orchestra and amateur theater, a high school band and numerous choirs; some of the best hockey players, figure skaters, and curlers in the country were our friends or classmates; there were three cinemas and half a dozen churches and numerous prosperous family businesses and several substantial hotels with formal dining rooms. Kirkland Lake was once the "Mile of Gold" with seven underground gold mines and a population that had peaked in the '60s at more than twenty thousand.

This summer, only one mine remains open, and the population of Kirkland Lake is about seven thousand. We know some people still: Wayne, an old school friend who had found us the place to stay; Judy, who took us all over Lake Kenogami in her party boat after midnight. Dave's

5

high school basketball coach came straight to me when we walked into the bar on Friday night and shook my hand and said what a good, gentle man Dave was. People from our time here know why we have come back. Memories are long and loyal. But most of those who stayed in the north no longer live in Kirkland Lake itself, with its small, dark houses from the '40s and '50s and dilapidated corner stores. They have built houses on the lakes nearby.

The town's center, the crooked, hilly main street called Government Road, is collapsing. This morning we silently observe the smallness and grubbiness and ground-down textures, the low self-esteem of the place, old, fat people who are shabby and unkempt and a little belligerent, unless they walk with their heads lowered. It is the Monday of a long weekend at the height of summer, but the streets are almost deserted.

It's a relief to get through town, across the railway tracks onto Highway 66 going east. Sara and I know every small hill, every bump and frost-heave and signpost on this thirteen-mile stretch of highway between Kirkland Lake and Dobie, upon which unraveled every significant journey of our childhoods. We are conscious of feeling emotionally detached from the town's human dramas (a depleted economy, tense squabbles about the bear hunt and whether or not to embrace the garbage from Toronto) but perfectly at home in the landscape—these trees (poplar, birch, mountain ash, and jack pine), and these shorelines (Gull Lake, Mud Lake—watch for moose in the swamp, then the lily-burdened marsh at the end of Crystal Lake), the sounds of this bush, the perfectly engineered curves of the roads, each outcrop of granite, the meadow where there are always blueberries, yes, today; it is the season.

JOHN DAVIS Botsford was born in the Kirkland Lake Hospital on April 28, 1949. Delivered, as all three of us were, by Dr. Tom Armstrong. People in small towns always know, or did then, who delivered them. Our parents were American: our father, Jack, came to northern Ontario as a mining engineer in the late '30s, served in the Royal Canadian Engineers, and returned to northern Michigan in 1946 to marry a young woman from his hometown. Our mother, Louise, visited Canada once before their marriage, and, famously in the family, Dad drove her quickly past the house where they would live only as he took her to the train station at the end of the visit. I was conceived during the camping trip that was their honeymoon journey, from Michigan to northern Ontario.

Dave (or Davy, as we called him until he married) was two years younger than me, and for the first few years of our lives we lived in that small pleasant house, unusual still in its sharply pointed roof over the porch, in the row of five staff houses on the Upper Canada Mine property, a row known as "the hill." The hill was about 2 kilometers from the village of Dobie, called "the townsite." Our childhood was contained by the gently rolling topography of a small piece of bush with a radius of about 5 or 6 kilometers: the hill, the townsite and the railway tracks and the reason for it all, Upper Canada Mine—a rambling mill for processing the gold, a water tower, modest offices, and the tarpaper-clad head frames over the two underground shafts (#1 and #2) about a kilometer apart. A circular network of gravel and tarred roads joined the mine, the hill, and the townsite, but there was only one road out to Highway 66, a bleak stretch of blacktop whose terminal points for us as children were Kirkland Lake to the west and the town of Rouyn-Noranda to the east on the Quebec border. Dobie and Upper Canada Mine were invisible from the highway, unsigned.

We experienced this scrubby landscape as dramatic and hilly; we went down to the townsite and back up to the hill. On the trail ("the shortcut") between the two were, then, to us and every other child, three distinct hills for tobogganing, and behind our house was another hill, thickly bushed, which gave way behind the house next door to a hill of soft yellow sand, deep enough in summer for the construction of elaborate towns and roads and large enough in winter for several ski trails. The bush looked impenetrable, but for children it was not. Like wild animals, we had a complex system of trails, and we named individual trees as signposts—the Witches' House, the Favorite Tree.

The townsite, Dobie, population around two hundred at best, was where mine employees lived, and where there were also, in the '50s, two general stores and a gas pump, a fire hall, one and briefly even two schools (one regular and one Catholic), and a shed with a woodstove beside the railway tracks, which curled in right beside the Rhamey house. Ontario Northland Railway trains would stop in front of the shed if the flag (a tattered white banner nailed to a pole) signaled them to do so. In winter, the shed provided shelter and warmth to members of the Beaverhouse First Nation, breaking their journey to or from their village on the lake and Kirkland Lake.

Dobie consisted of three streets, unnamed then. The houses were known by the names of their inhabitants: Rhamey, Ford, Sceviour, Nystrand, Drury, Barney, Meaniss, McDougall, Kublas, Piekarz, Starcevich, Lamontagne. Except on the middle street, all the houses backed onto the bush, stuccoed and tarpapered bungalows or frail little frame houses on their own wells.

Sara was born in 1951. I went with my parents to the hospital in Kirkland Lake to bring her home; I remember sitting in the back seat of the car and my mother holding Sara tightly in the front seat. I was wearing a pale yellow dress with puffed sleeves and lace trim and matching bloomers with rows of white lace stitched on the back, but I was wearing them backward, as our babysitter did not know that the lace ruffles were meant to decorate my bottom. I was allowed, carefully and proudly, to hold on my lap the metal tray of glass bottles filled with formula. We were not breastfed, as formula was the nutritious, hygienic choice of informed women in the '50s. As a consequence, we were all chubby as small children; Pablum and tapioca pudding and generous helpings of milk and cheese were also contributing factors. I was known as the Campbell Kid or Apple Ass. Sara thought her middle name was Fatbottom. Our parents had a sardonic sense of humor, which we all inherited.

That same year a new house was built for us at the end of the row on the hill—the manager's house, as our father had worked his way up the mine's hierarchy to the top staff position. As soon as the snow was collapsing into rivulets in the ditches that spring, Davy (sturdy, with bright red curls, pale blue eyes, and a robust nature) and I gravely walked down the gravel road every morning after breakfast and sat side by side on a heap of bulldozed dirt to watch the building of the house. When we moved in, we insisted on carrying down our prized possessions, especially his yellow tractor and the box of wooden blocks (between us, each with one hand curled through the handles). This watchfulness—absorbing myriad technical details, filing them in some rational order so that they could always be accessed—was a trait Dave acquired from Dad, but unlike Dad, Dave understood how to build things and how engines and electricity worked. I have no doubt he remembered for a lifetime tiny details of that construction, just as he always knew the make, model, and color of every car that our family owned, and the size of the motors on the outboards up at Beaverhouse or out at Crystal. These things framed his imagination.

My memory of such things is casual and desultory, because I did not value the artifacts themselves. I remember the smocking on my dresses and elaborate birthday cakes built by our mother (a train for Davy, a doll in a turquoise icing ballgown for me) and learning to read when I was four at the breakfast room table (*Down, down, down*), and my mother's index finger tapping hard into my right shoulder when I was practicing the piano. In winter, the deep etchings of Jack Frost on my bedroom window and our father's deliberate ritual of draining the radiators into Mason jars, always at night, sitting on the edge of my bed with a cigarette in his mouth. The smell of my father as I watched him shave. In summer, lying on the lawn in my bathing suit in the afternoon, as close as possible to Rocky, the biddable black-and-white springer spaniel, watching the clouds drift overhead. In autumn, the three of us diving into fragrant piles of leaves we'd so carefully raked up just minutes before, burying ourselves in separate piles and whispering to one another through garden hoses like walkie-talkies.

We loved our new house. It was white, two-storied, grand by local standards, with a pillared porch, green shutters, and a green roof. It was set back against the bush, and the lawn was studded with clumps of white birch and a stand of large spruce trees. The backyard attracted a host of birds—evening and pine grosbeaks, yellow-shafted flickers and blue jays—and flying squirrels, and regularly in spring, a few scrawny black bears came over the hill to paw at the garbage cans. The rolling front lawn would over time acquire flower beds overflowing with sweet peas and begonias during the short, longed-for summers. Our family lived here for twenty years.

The interior layout of the house was balanced and spacious, a source of deep if obscure satisfaction to all of us, it turned out. There was a vestibule and a square front hall from which a staircase led to the second floor. To the right of the hall, an archway opened onto the dining room and kitchen, with a breakfast room off the kitchen; to the left

11

of the hall, a living room ran the length of the house, with a fireplace, bookshelves, and a place for the upright piano. A back hall joined the living room to the kitchen, and it contained three doors on one side—a large closet, stairs to the basement, and a powder room—on the other, the back door to outside. This made the ground floor into an open, circular track, a dynamic space for chases and hide-and-seek. That same design was echoed in the basement: playroom–furnace room–corridor–sewing room–playroom. Upstairs, there was a bathroom and four bedrooms and a hallway in which there was barely room for a small bookcase filled with encyclopedias purchased from a traveling salesman and years of *National Geographic* magazines.

When I visited Dobie twenty years after leaving home, I was astounded at how tiny the house was, how small the rooms, how narrow that back hall, as it had instilled in me very grand ideas of proportion and scale in a living space. The three hills on the shortcut—where we tobogganed after dark and came bursting home red-cheeked in wet snowsuits for sloppy joes and cocoa in the breakfast room with our friends—were not hills at all, more like the modulations of a streambed.

12

I RECALL childhood to the age of ten as a time when there were clear-cut rituals, things that were always done the same way, the days and weeks defined by activity and task and season. Our father left for the mine every day by seven, after making his own breakfast and a pot of strong, percolated coffee—which got stronger as the morning and the years wore on—for Louise, our mother. He came home for lunch most days, and after listening to the CBC news at one, took his nap on the chesterfield in the living room until exactly one-thirty, when he went back to the mine. He wore a shirt and tie every day, except when he went underground, to examine a particular stope, to discuss the opening of a new level, to compare elaborate engineering drawings with the rock face, or maybe just for the pleasure of riding down in the gently swaying cage with all the men in their boots and hard hats and then entering the absolute darkness of a drift. He loved more than anything to go underground. He returned home at six, read the papers in his chair, drank a tall glass of sharp, malty beer in the early days. We were usually allowed one sip. From June until October, he would spend an hour every evening working in his vegetable garden and then have his beer. He brought home the *Globe and Mail* every day, and also got the *Northern Daily News* and the *Northern Miner* and *Time* magazine but never the *Telegraph* or *Star*. Sara and I read the *Globe and Mail* on our stomachs on the living room floor for years, a habit our mother did not care for.

Our mother's days were intensely busy when we were small children; she had terrific energy and a strong sense of household management. She cooked and baked and did whatever had to be done with fruits and vegetables in season. Dad had carved his garden out of the impossible marshy bush across the road from the house, and it produced a surprising quantity of carrots, green beans, broccoli, cauliflower, cabbage, and squash for freezing, preserving, or storing over winter. Mom's mornings were mostly for cooking and the afternoons for sewing. She had a special room in the basement, much admired by other women and by the children who came to play and the relatives who visited from Michigan. There was a long red Formica counter for cutting out patterns. A bank of bottomless drawers for fabric, patterns, and sewing supplies. A deep sink, a sewing machine (first a treadle Singer and later an electric version), a large mangle iron for sheets and pillowcases and tablecloths, the ironing board, washer, dryer. A cold room against the outside wall at the far end, with shelves for preserves, big bins for keeping root vegetables over winter, and the freezer. A laundry chute (I thought of it as the laundry *shoot*) that passed through the house, from the upstairs bathroom through the kitchen into a large basket in the basement. This was the most ingenious feature of our house, and it was surely her idea.

I doubt that our mother had to refer to magazines like *Chatelaine* or *Good Housekeeping* for her sense of order. She had studied and taught nursing and home economics in Michigan before marrying and moving to the Canadian bush. Homemaking was her profession, and as long as that could be her occupation, it was. (This sense of purpose began to unravel when we became teenagers.) She was an excellent cook—everyone said so—one who entertained generously, and she made all of our clothes (a badge of honor). She never sewed for herself but purchased her wardrobe from a couple of dress shops locally, and once a year, before the Prospectors' Convention, she would have outfits (dresses, suits,

14

handbags, and hats) sent up on approval by train from "The Room" at Simpsons in Toronto. She had a strong sense of community: she taught Sunday school before the United Church services in Dobie, belonged to the Ladies' Aid, and later joined the hospital auxiliary in Kirkland Lake.

Much of Mom's creative energy went into the making of our clothes; her sewing room was an atelier. Our play was frequently interrupted by the tedious task of being fitted, standing with suddenly itchy legs on the long counter when we were really small, and then on a chair, Mom turning us like chickens roasting on a spit, pinning armpits and waists and collars and hems. She did not just sew for us; she knitted and smocked. (It is our naptime, and the house is silent, and Mom has set up her smocking board on the dining room table. The light falls over her shoulder. Pinned to the board is the bodice of a pale pink, polished cotton dress for me, with threads of contrasting shades puckered and pulled into an intricate pattern. She looks up and smiles at me when I come down the stairs.)

Every day had assigned tasks and rituals. Groceries were phoned into the big Italian grocery store on Wednesday and delivered on Friday afternoon. Milk was delivered in glass bottles daily to the back door. Spic and Span Cleaners came to the front door; dry cleaning was picked up in bundles on Tuesday and brought back in long paper sleeves on Friday. There was no postman; the mail came to the mine office, and Dad brought it home at suppertime. Some of these rituals changed as we got older and our scheduled activities altered things, so I remember Thursday as both a music lesson day and later a town day. On town days Mom drove into Kirkland Lake to shop, go to the library, have her hair done. I loved to go with her, into Kresge's past the soda fountain, or up the broad staircase into the more formal lay-out of Eaton's, then to the little Singer sewing shop for pat-terns and notions, into Eddie Duke's photography shop to pick up camera supplies for our father, into Trussler's Hard-ware, and finally, I always hoped, into Emile's Bakery at the far end of Government Road for a French pastry. These trips were privileges for me as the eldest; Sara and Davy would have a babysitter.

Friday was cleaning day, when either Mrs. Piekarz or Mrs. Lamontagne came for the day and worked in tandem with Mom. Then she drove them home with an overflowing basket of laundry for ironing. Friday was also the day that Mom baked bread and made large batches of vegetable soup and casseroles to freeze or big, open bowls of applesauce and tapioca pudding that we children always tried to get a dessertspoon into when we came home from school, while it was still warm in the fridge. Saturday was spaghetti night, meaning a rich bolognaise sauce and garlic bread and a huge salad with her dressing of Roquefort cheese, red-wine vinegar, and caraway seeds. Sunday was Sunday school and church, lunch of pea soup, and then roast beef dinner (rare roast beef, broccoli with a cheese sauce).

During the week we ate supper together at the round wooden table in the breakfast room, in our allotted places. We always sat in the same places at either that table or the dining room table, where we ate Sunday dinner, with the Royal Doulton china, the only time that Dad muttered a blessing. Our family dramas, major and minor, large and small, unfolded at the table. It was where we discussed subjects like Diefenbaker and Elvis Presley and bomb shelters and good manners and the habits of flying squirrels, and where we children were encouraged to debate with our father, who took up outrageous positions just to provoke us. It was also where important announcements were made about plans for family trips or relatives coming to visit, and where we children were told things that somehow we had to be told as a group, things our parents had agreed beforehand were important or sensitive.

One Sunday, we three children went with our mother to church at the school in the townsite, as usual. This day our father drove us down, which was not usual, but he didn't stay. When he came back to drive us home after church, they no doubt exchanged silent glances in the front seat. Then Mom went straight to the kitchen to prepare the after-church lunch of Habitant pea soup and her corn bread (which we called johnnycake), freshly made that morning before church.

When she called us to the table, there was a smell of burned soup. Mom never burned food, and she was crying uncontrollably. We three were alarmed by this and determined to eat the soup anyway. We sat in our chairs around the breakfast room table, white Wedgwood bowls of charred soup before us. "Would you pass the johnnycake, dear?" asked our father. She did not speak, sobbing openly as she passed the plate of johnnycake, first to me on her right. We all loved johnnycake, and there was a contented flurry of passing the butter, breaking and buttering our pieces. At least she could see that the johnnycake was fine.

Our father picked up, then set down his soup spoon and cleared his throat. His voice was gentle, as it could be on occasion. "I'm afraid," he said, "that something happened sometime during the night last night. Or early this morning."

"What?" I asked sharply, on our behalf, my voice in a higher register than usual. Our mother dared not look at any of us children. Sara was pale. Davy was silent.

"Rocky—" Dad had only just begun, but all three of us suddenly realized our springer spaniel was not there. That we had not seen him that morning. That the house was very quiet.

"He must've been chasing cars, on the road to the townsite. He was run over . . . "

"I'm sure he died instantly, he didn't suffer . . . " said our mother.

"Where?" I blurted.

"Across from Filmores'," said Dad. "He was found in the ditch, early this morning. Somebody called the mine—"

This last was drowned out by a harsh cry, followed by big gulping sobs, from Davy, who stared at our parents with stricken, juicing eyes and his mouth wide open, filled with johnnycake.

It was one of the few times that Sara and I saw Davy cry as a child. It was also one of the few times that Dad did not ask us if we were bleeding, his usual response to crying. We were stuck in our places, no one saying anything more, politely eating scorched soup and crying.

DAVY WAS the enigmatic, perplexing child. Until he was five, he was jolly and healthy. But something happened then, or more than one thing: he was playing in the shallow water on the sandy beach of Larder Lake, when a large, noisy motorboat drove straight toward him, only swinging away at the last minute. This incident left him terrified of water for some years. Also around this time, he suffered an illness with a very high fever, after which he was never chubby again and at times was very thin. Was this scarlet fever, rheumatic fever, meningitis? It seems odd to me that I don't know and neither did he. Did these two events in combination exert a lingering trauma, and was this sickness a seed that would erupt many years later?

He had myriad little illnesses and anxieties. He got stomachaches and sore ears. He thought his feet were not straight, his arms too long. He worried about his very thick, curly hair falling out and would compulsively pull at it looking for clumps. As a small boy, he would not say the number 17 when counting. He had arbitrary routines, eating one food group on his plate completely before tackling the next. He had sticking points: piano practice, which he hated; long pants, which he wanted long before he got them.

Dancing lessons: both Davy and I took dancing lessons weekly in Kirkland Lake for several years. I took ballet, Davy took tap, and we carried our dance shoes in purple Seagram's bags into the basement studio on Government Road. Davy hated these lessons and especially the graduation recital on the stage of the Strand Theatre, in costumes sewn by Mom. There are photos of me as a serene raindrop in pale green taffeta and Davy as a glowering railway conductor in a striped jacket, carrying a dented cardboard suitcase. He threw a howling, red-faced tantrum backstage before the recital and had to be forced onto the stage, where he cried throughout his number including the stiff little bow at the end.

His emotional connections were compromised by being a shy, quiet boy between two girls. He was always profoundly bashful in the company of adults and strangers. He would refuse to greet people even when prompted to do so. Within the family he was not timid but incapable of expressing emotions other than anger. His anger surfaced when he was teased, as he was relentlessly by Sara and her friends because they knew they could goad him into a rage for which he would get into trouble, not them. He always owned up if he did something wrong. Our parents also teased him, possibly as part of a manliness campaign. In the car, Mom would pretend to know the names of cows along the roadside, and he would sulk in frustration when she would not tell him *how* she knew their names.

His one sign of vulnerability was a ginger-colored bear named Teddy Bear, his constant companion. If he had anything daring or serious or heartfelt to say he would hold the bear up in front of his face and speak from behind it: *Mummy, Teddy said* shit; *Teddy wants to go home now; Teddy is really sorry*... Mom and Sara and I would also be able to convey feelings or ideas to Davy through Teddy. The bear was much stitched and darned and tenderly restuffed over the years by Mom, who also made him a pair of corduroy overalls that kept him in one piece (and in Dave's possession) for almost 45 years.

DAVY WAS only happy if he was building something or if he was in the bush.

The bush was our playground. From a very young age, we were sent out to play right after breakfast, in winter in thickly padded snowsuits with scarves tied over our mouths, and in spring and summer and fall with a paperbag lunch of egg or peanut butter sandwiches, cookies and fruit, and chocolate milk in a Coke bottle. We went straight up the hill behind the house into the bush, where we had dozens of trails and caves and hiding places. We squatted beside the road digging drains through the mud. We packed trails in the snow and built elaborate houses, with rooms and doorways and benches and chairs carved of snow. We learned to skate on a field beside the curling club, where a rough rink was plowed out inside a ring of high snowbanks and watered into smooth ice. Here we spent hours as young children, first with our parents (on weekend afternoons, our mother in her huge beaver coat, pushing us along on little black learner skates) and then with all the children from the hill and Dobie, after school, late on Friday night when the ice was lit by a string of bare lightbulbs, and all day Saturday and Sunday after church. We warmed ourselves, and flirted and squabbled, in the Snake Room, so called because the skin of a garter snake was stretched over an opening behind the counter, through which we eavesdropped on the adults, curling and drinking on the other side. When we were a little older there were certain beaver ponds back in the bush that suddenly became small rinks on cold, still winter days, when the weather was exactly right to create a hard polished surface.

In summer we played in the sandbox and in the sand pit behind the Cheeseman house next door and in the screen-house in spring (safe from bears and blackflies). In fine weather all year round we would be expected to stay outside until midafternoon, at least. We told time by the signals from the mine—the noon whistle, the end-of-shift sirens, and the rumble of the miners' bus changing gears on the hilly gravel road between the two head frames.

THERE IS a photo of the three of us when we were quite small, sitting on an overturned canoe, at Crystal Lake. We always had a canoe. Our father taught us to paddle, a skill honed at the summer camps we went to from the age of twelve. As a family, he made sure that we explored and knew well the rivers and lakes around Dobie and Kirkland Lake and east into northern Quebec. We were piled into a big outboard motorboat and taken up Lake Beaverhouse for overnight camping trips, when we all slept together in what now seems a very small canvas tent from the war. We fished, from shore and in canoes and rowboats. We learned to skeet-shoot at a site set up behind Number Two shaft at the mine. Davy was taught to use guns, first a BB gun and then a rifle, and by the time he was a teenager, he was a hunter, with his own gun and his Labrador retriever, Beaverhouse Chief. He and his friends went for weekend camping trips to remote lakes as soon as one of them had a driver's license.

In the autumn, as we became old enough, we each walked alone through the bush with our father, who carried a rifle or a shotgun, ostensibly hunting for partridge or moose or deer. I never saw an animal killed on these occasions, but I am sure that Davy did. I experienced these walks as a rare chance to be alone with my father, when he would name trees and birds and lecture me about rocks and show me how to look for tracks, and I would stand silently, happily, beside him in a clearing as he smoked a cigarette and pondered.

Our father was a handsome man, tall, lean, with dark brown eyes and a prominent widow's peak (a sign of beauty, he told us with a glimmer of a smile, along with his long "Plantagenet" toe). Distant and preoccupied, as was the custom for fathers then. Stern; it was he who meted out discipline on instruction from Mom, and we were afraid of him. We craved his fleeting moments of tenderness and demonstrations of love, which was how we read being alone with

23

him in the bush or his sharing with us his knowledge, or those times when his voice would soften and his eyes would become shiny. We learned how to match his mordant wit, to make him laugh, and then we watched in adoration as a twinkle appeared in his eyes and they would literally turn up at the corners.

He taught us to ski. We would follow him, on his long, slim hand-carved hickory skis on powdery trails through the sunlit bush behind the house and around the mine, until we were confident enough to ski on our own. Then we stamped out our own hills behind the house. Several winters we made large ski hills in the bush between Dobie and Crystal Lake; we took sandwiches and hot cocoa in thermoses and skied out along the power line and spent the entire day packing hills and skiing down them until the snow was tinted pink by the setting sun. Davy was always in charge of skiing expeditions and the design of our ski hills.

Until I went to university, we three skied together at little ski clubs around Dobie like Swastika and Larder Lake, with the most basic facilities and rope tows, and the slightly larger ones, Raven Mountain and Mont Kanasuta, with T-bar lifts and more challenging slopes. Davy and Sara were more athletic and physically courageous than I was. (My most disappointing Christmas was when I was twelve, the one where I was sure that I was getting skis because I was finally no longer an invalid with acute nephritis. On Christmas morning my heart leapt when I detected the outline of skis behind a curtain beside the tree. But they were for Davy or Sara; I got a puffy, pale pink quilted housecoat, which I loathed forever.) I loved to ski with Davy; he was able to teach me and give me courage to make up for what I lacked in skill. I could stand at the top of Raven Mountain forever, unless Davy was there to lead me down.

For several winters, Davy constructed a ski jump near the bottom of the hill behind our house. He would practice jumping for hours by himself, over and over and over. One bitterly cold and dark afternoon, I came home on the bus from high school to find him lying almost unconscious, face down on the floor, Sara, small and white-faced, sitting beside him, our mother probably at a meeting in town. He had fallen during a jump and broken his leg. He had dragged himself over the snow from the hill, several hundred meters, inch by inch, through the back door and up two steps into the kitchen. But he did not cry.

In retrospect, it seems remarkable how much freedom we had as children to roam the bush, a range of miles and miles, crisscrossed with train tracks, power lines, soft, sandy lumbering roads. Our parents had no apparent anxiety about our playing on abandoned mine sites and in the foundations of old houses and mining camps. Walking the railway tracks all the way to town, putting our ear to the steel to hear trains, climbing forest fire lookouts back in the bush. Clambering over piles of discarded diamond drill core and daring one another to walk across the remnants of the cage supports over deserted mine shafts. The snow houses became villages far back in the bush, and later there were forts and then two-story tree forts made mostly by the boys; those I never saw, in clearings where Davy and his friends built campfires and brought their dogs and rifles and slept overnight.

A Kirkland Lake man reminisced a few years ago in a northern magazine about "the Botsford children" playing softball on the expanse of pale, solidified mine waste behind the Upper Canada mill that we called the slimes; I don't remember that. I recall that the slimes were off-limits, because of quicksand and bears. But I don't remember many other rules about the bush. Except for when we were very small, I do not remember our play being supervised at all. It was our only form of wildness in otherwise orderly, well-dressed, even regimented lives.

IN BAD weather and once it got dark, we descended to our playroom in the basement. This was a serious, orderly place with a painted concrete floor and a sewage pipe that ran like a stripper's pole through the center of the low room. Here we had our big box of polished blocks, made by the mine carpenter, Earl Fagan, who also made the dollhouse exactly like our house, with a roof and sides that came off, and soft furnishings made by Mom from scraps of curtains and slip-covers in our real house. We had Plasticine and finger paints and, later, hula hoops. We had many books (but no comic books—these we read furtively when we visited friends in the townsite). There was a record player and a huge pile of 45s and 78s. We knew all the words to songs like "Bibbity

Bobbety Boo" and "Mairzy Doats" and "Lucky, Lucky, Lucky Me." We pirouetted to "Swan Lake" and scared ourselves in the dark with the Painted Desert movement of the "Grand Canyon Suite." No television until we were all teenagers; our parents disapproved of the "boob tube."

Sara and I had a succession of dolls, with clothes, including bonnets, mittens, and bootees, made by Mom. Davy had a cupboard full of Dinky cars and trucks that came from the United Cigar Store. He played incessantly with the Tinker Toys and Meccano set, but we all built things together. He spent long hours at Dad's workbench in the furnace room—planing wood, sawing, making little boats and houses, whatever he could fashion from pieces of scrap lumber. He built a small pool table when he was about ten, and one summer a series of stilts for Sara and him that got taller and taller, so tall that they had to climb onto the garage roof to get onto them. We had elaborate projects that we would work on together over days or weeks, and they always had stories or plots; the stilts turned Davy and Sara into circus performers; we set up hospitals in the garage and secret clubhouses in a neighbor's basement. We became a band, with a washboard (strummed with Mom's thimbles on our fingers), a comb covered in tissue paper, and Dad's gut bucket (a washtub upside down, with a string attached to it and to a broomstick so that it could be plucked like a bass) and played along with records or sang songs like "Georgia Brown" and "I've Been Workin' on the Railroad," the songs our parents sang raucously at house

27

parties. We harmonized wildly and did jazzy improvs and what we did not know was called scat singing.

One Saturday afternoon before Mother's Day, we were in the basement agonizing over what to give our mother as a present. (We did not have pocket money or an allowance until we were teenagers.) I was probably on the couch with a book. Davy would be fiddling with some pieces of wood by the open furnace room door. Sara would be sitting on Mom's sewing counter, legs swinging furiously.

"We have to make her something," I said.

"What?" Davy said.

"Build something . . . " said Sara.

"Like what?" Davy looked at me.

"I know," I said. "What about my little cross! You could make a platform for it, like an altar! And then Sara and I'll decorate it."

"I'd have to paint it first," said Davy, already looking for wood and an open can of paint.

"What's an altar?" asked Sara, looking dubious.

"It's what they have in real churches for crosses; you'll see." I snuck up to my bedroom and brought down the cross in my pocket. It was a plain white cross, not a crucifix, standing on a ledge of narrow steps, about three inches high and made of a plastic that glowed in the dark. I was inexplicably fond of this relic, probably given to me by a Catholic babysitter; I used to hold it when I went to sleep, soothed by the eerie greenish light that filtered through the skin of my hand. (Sara still has this cross on her dressing table.)

Davy nailed some scrap pieces of two-by-four into a three-tiered platform. He sanded it and painted it pale green and hid it behind a box under the workbench. The next day after church and lunch we hurried down to the basement. Davy glued the cross onto the top step of his platform. Sara and I decorated the platform with small white candles (the ones from the brass Christmas ornament with the whirling angels) and draped a string of pale pink artificial flowers (left over from an Easter floral arrangement) around the cross and its base. We were all enormously pleased by this artifact.

At twilight, our parents were in the living room, in their respective chairs, reading. Mom was also knitting.

"Sara, go upstairs and turn out the lights and tell them there's a surprise," I said. "Davy, go into the kitchen and get the matches."

We assembled, whispering, in the back hall. I held the altar, Davy lit the candles, and the three of us solemnly paraded into the living room, a priestess and two acolytes.

"Holy, Holy, Holy, Lord God Almighty," we sang softly, reverently; it was the song about the Trinity, the first piece in the United Church hymnal. Mom and Dad sat, just as solemnly, in their chairs as we approached with our Mother's Day offering.

Religion for us as children was more a form of theater than an expression of faith. We were not a devout family at all, but from a young age we recognized the power of religious symbols and ceremonies. Mom took the three of us

29

to the Dobie schoolhouse every Sunday for a service led by a harried United Church minister whose parish also included real churches in Larder Lake and Virginiatown. I sang in the choir, which rehearsed with Mrs. Sceviour every Thursday evening. Sometimes, on special occasions, Mom and I went into Kirkland Lake to the real United Church there. When I was a teenager I sang solos in church, songs like "The Lord's Prayer," "Oh Holy Night," and "Bless this house, oh Lord we pray, make it safe by night and day . . . " I also knew by heart the Roman Catholic chants—" . . . blessed art thou among women and blessed is the fruit of thy womb, Jesus . . . "—from listening to a program called *The Rosary* on the radio. Our father often made us sit as a family completely silent during Sunday dinner, listening to Billy Graham's sermons just because he loved his voice and rich rhetoric. It seemed natural to know all the words to many hymns and carols and to kneel beside our beds nightly, to say our prayers, "Now I lay me down to sleep . . . ," even as we understood somehow that our parents did not have anything that might be called faith. So, on Christmas mornings, we three would get up between four and five and go whispering into the bathroom and huddle together under a blanket in the dark on the floor, softly singing carols because the bathroom acoustics gave us pleasure. And because we wanted to make the Christmas morning rituals begin.

When I was eleven, I experimented seriously with faith because I was ill, confined to my bed for almost eight months with a kidney infection. For months I listened carefully to *The Rosary* and *Hymn Sing* on the radio, and one spring Sunday afternoon I used a wide, pink grosgrain hair ribbon to lash together two two-by-twos into a cross, which I planted in the bush at the edge of the backyard. As a teenager I would sneak into the back of the French Roman Catholic church in Kirkland Lake and breathe in the smell of candles and incense and stare at the Stations of the Cross and feel that I was missing something. I don't know if Davy or Sara had a similar religious crisis, but if they did we never talked about it. They stopped going to church long before I did. My sense is that Davy, especially, only found spiritual meaning in the wilderness.

THE IMPOSED disciplines of our childhood included household chores—shoveling snow, raking leaves, and sweeping the walks, helping in Dad's vegetable garden by cutting black tarpaper collars for the cabbages and pounding sauerkraut in the fall, activities thought by our parents to be instructional as well as useful—and dance and piano lessons, Brownies and Cubs, homework, church. From the age of six, we all took piano lessons, practicing every morning before school; my shift was the first, from six o'clock, then Davy, then Sara. We also practiced after school every day. Sara and I took Royal Conservatory exams and played in Kiwanis music festivals until the end of high school, as she and I were outgoing, at ease before strangers, and always performers; Davy adamantly was not. Davy was allowed to stop piano lessons early, when it appeared he had no aptitude except for improvisation and because he simply refused to play in public. (He really wanted to play the drums, and I wanted to be a drum majorette like Nancy Tully up the road, but we were not allowed to pursue these interests.)

Davy and I excelled at Cubs and Brownies; I was ready to fly up, as they said, to Girl Guides, but there were none in Dobie, and that was the year I was sick in bed with a kidney infection. Davy thrived on skills like firebuilding and tent-pitching and orienteering and was chosen as best Wolf Cub at a jamboree in Kirkland Lake one year. He did not tell us this. I remember when we found out—because the cubmaster gave Dad a photograph at the office—we were very surprised and inordinately pleased.

OUR CHILDHOOD was recorded in photographs. Dad had a darkroom and was a good amateur photographer for years, although his interest subsided as cameras became more sophisticated and color slides became common. I have many of Dad's pictures of me and Davy as infants and also formal, hand-tinted photographs taken by a professional photographer. These portraits were taken in Dobie in a rooming house run by a slightly scary old lady named Mrs. Urino, who was toothless but grinned always and made delicious cabbage rolls and for a time bred chinchillas. All of these details hang over the yellowing photographs like an aura. I remember the room, and being posed on a high table covered with a soft beige cloth. Davy was two, holding a red ball, in white shoes and socks and pale blue shorts and white blouse. I was four, in a smocked, reddish-rust dress, with a matching fat satin hair ribbon.

It is clear from photographs that our dress code was stringent, with everything including our coats and hats made by Mom. Our clothes always matched. If I had a plaid skirt (kilt-style), Davy had plaid shorts with matching suspenders, and we both had black vests and white blouses— mine had a puffed sleeve; Davy's was straight. In early school photos, we were dressed alike: navy sweaters, me in buttoned pointed collar; Davy, open; Sara, rounded. Sara and I had white gloves and purses. I had a white rabbit muff, and we all had parkas with fox-trimmed hoods. Our wardrobe was partly determined by women's magazines, McCall pattern books and Eaton's catalogues, but our clothes were distinctive because Mom had a sense of style unlike that of anyone else's mother. She took pride in this. We were ambivalent, self-conscious about our bonnets and matching colors and embarrassed as we got older, because we wanted to look like everyone else. Especially Davy, who was mortified by his tucked-in shirts and little ties and short pants. He increasingly sought identity in the ordinariness of the townsite boys.

We had clothes for each season, stored in off-seasons in the basement, in mothball-reeking chests in the corridor between Mom's sewing room and Dad's furnace room. This same corridor was where the sauerkraut fermented every autumn and where we played hide-and-seek, burrowing into our mother's fragrant dresses, which hung at one end of the hallway, or our father's scratchy, woolen outer garments, at the furnace room end. The furnace room was where Dad stored his guns and ammunition and the big trunk that held his army uniform and trombone and where he had his fully equipped darkroom (off-limits for hide-and-seek).

Dad took photos of the three of us together, one or two every year until we were in our early teens. Mom would dress us in matching outfits, and we would pose, or rather be posed by Mom, for Dad, in front of the house, on the porch, in the road framed by snow-covered trees. On a toboggan, under the birch trees. I smiled, pleasantly if unmemorably, in these pictures; Davy grimaced with painful shyness and Sara (who always had a larger-than-life character) mugged or howled and had to be placated with a banana.

The final group photograph was a lugubrious studio portrait I organized when I was fifteen, with Eddie Duke, the professional photographer in Kirkland Lake, and paid for myself as a surprise for Mom and Dad. It is a horrible picture; we are plain, pale, and smiling grimly, and Davy's hair is very short, but at least our clothes are no longer matching. By then we were all going to school in Kirkland Lake and our personas were more our own than our parents'.

34   UNTIL THE sixth grade, we went to the one-room schoolhouse in Dobie. Her Majesty the Queen presided from a photograph over the blackboard, and the only beautiful, mysterious object in the room was a brass and wood replica of the solar system that sat on top of the piano. We had a succession of single-women teachers but never a man; the school inspector was always a man. The grades were set up in rows running from front to back, and spelling tests were done in grade order: grade one: *cat*. Grade two: *house*.

Grade three . . . and so on. Coats, scarves, hats, and mittens were hung in the cloakroom, boots neatly placed beneath our designated hooks. There were two smelly toilets in the basement and a sink with cold running water and a dribbling water fountain there as well. We did not much care for the school basement, except at Halloween, when it became an elaborate haunted house.

Sara and I spent only five years in this school, because we both skipped a grade; Davy did not. This did not seem to trouble him; girls were more likely to skip than boys, and by then he had his precious cohort of male friends all in the same grade. It was a place where we quickly learned the rules of society, the strict hierarchy of age, the cruelties of gangs of the slightly older and taller taunting the younger and smaller. The dramas of insults like "Liar, liar pants on fire," and bloodied noses and broken toys. The tensions that sometimes erupted between the townsite and Snob Hill— so-called when there were fights. The Dobie school ground was a rough-and-tumble place and sometimes a test of family loyalties against peer pressure. For a while there was a big, complicated game called Crows and Eagles that engaged all twenty or so children every recess, with elaborate rules about foraging for imaginary food and fighting and taking captives outside the boundaries of carefully demarcated corners of the school ground that were "home-free" nests. Once in this melee, Sara was chased by the biggest boy in the school, Cecil Meaniss, who threw her on the ground and pounded her back until she cried. Davy saw this, helpless and scared, but after school he waited for Sara and walked

home with her, pushing her bicycle. We knew we were supposed to look out for one another.

We walked home every day for lunch, up the shortcut
and back again, even in the dead of winter. A perfect, perfect
winter day was when we could walk across the crust through
the bush to school. This day was heralded by a bright sun-
rise and all the smoke from the houses in the townsite running together in a straight line along the horizon. But an
even better day was the morning in spring when we could
finally ride our bicycles to school. That day came after the
snow had really melted and after the mud had subsided on
the sides of the road. That day came with the appearance
in the bush of soft ground pine and the pale pink, sweet-
smelling trailing arbutus. I fell off my bike every spring on
the one curve on the hill going down to school, but Davy
and Sara rarely fell. Sara was a restless tomboy; Davy just did
all those things carefully and well. Riding bikes and scabby
knees and trailing arbutus are fused in my memory.

DURING SCHOOL holidays and in the summers, we traveled
a great deal as a family. Our parents were determined to
show us that there were places other than northern Ontario.
We went to Niagara Falls and to Washington, D.C., to visit
our father's brother and his family. We took the overnight
train to Toronto, where we got off the train early in the morning and went directly *under* the street to the dining room
at the Royal York Hotel, where we ate oatmeal and brown
sugar and thick cream with heavy silver spoons. It was in

the lobby of the Royal York Hotel that our father famously announced, loudly and to our intense mortification, Now we will *all* go to the bathroom. This phrase became a family mantra that we would say in unison thereafter.

We went to Florida by train one winter to visit our grandparents. The new experiences on this trip were intense and many. They included spaghetti dinner in a second-floor restaurant near the train station in Philadelphia, where the waiter wrapped large cloth napkins under our chins. And our first motel, a pink stucco place right on a beach at Clearwater, Florida, and swimming in salt water. Huge grapefruits, warm from the sun and not ever in the fridge, and oranges and lemons growing on trees, and a balmy softness in the air that was a combination of the ocean and flowering trees and sensual warm breezes in March, of all things.

These journeys were important to the fabric of our family life. They reinforced the closeness of us three as children and somehow, because of the small and particular nature of the exoticisms, underlined the isolation of growing up in the bush of northern Ontario. Nobody else in Dobie ever left Dobie for such magical destinations.

When we traveled by car, we sang, all five of us, with great gusto and wonderful cacophony, because Sara and I were the only ones who could carry a tune. We sang rounds—"Row, Row, Row Your Boat" and "Three Blind Mice" and "Frère Jacques." We sang "Alouett-ah, jaunty Alouett-ah." Our mother always started, "There were ten in the bed and the little one said, Roll over, roll over! They all rolled over and one fell out." We three vigorously acted this out in the back seat. Our father's repertoire included "Oh My Darling, Darling Clementine," for which he knew many verses, a song about ham and eggs in a boarding house, and his party piece, which he sang in an ersatz Cockney accent: "Eneree the Hayth Oi Yam, Oi Yam." It went: "I got married to the widow next door; she'd been married seven times before and everyone was an Eneree (ENEREE! We all shouted here). She wouldn't have a Willie or a Sam. I'm 'er eighth old man called Eneree (ENEREE!) Eneree the Hayth Oi Yam."

Sara's and my crowning achievement as a car song was an exquisitely harmonized version of "Climb Every Mountain," which we will still sing on exceptional occasions, by request.

Davy had a couple of quiet songs that he would sing alone, both about logging: "Oh, I'm a lumberjack and I'm okay..." And one he made up: "Haul away the woods, haul away the woods..." Also in the car, Davy conducted muttered auctions in a nasal monotone into his baseball mitt, which the rest of us always found extremely amusing.

The three of us had elaborate car games and forms of mutual torture with names that meant something only to the family: pimpling; mushy-gee-gee; up doh-doh, down, down, down. (Pimpling was the worst sibling insult; it meant pointing an elbow into someone's face and glaring, and it was called pimpling because a pointed elbow resembled a breast, which we referred to as a pimple. "Mummy, Marian's pimpling me!" "Marian, stop pimpling Davy...")

In summer, we went every year until I was 15 to northern Michigan to visit relatives. We loved these trips, the
being there if not the actual journey, which was 500 miles
over roads that were awful until we got to Michigan, where
they were smooth and lined with woods, not bush. Mostly
this was Mom and the three of us. We always stopped at the
same places en route and ate the same food. We had road
contests: Twenty Questions, I Spy, and the first to see Castle
Rock near St. Ignace, the first to see the statue of Paul Bunyan. When we got to Petoskey, Michigan, we went to a particular hamburger place for supper, and then Mom changed
our matching clothes in the bathrooms and brushed our
hair and scrubbed our faces so that we looked perfect for
our arrival at our grandmother's house in the village of Central Lake in Antrim County.

Our mother was deeply ambivalent about these trips,
especially about her own mother, with whom she was
trapped for her entire life in a cage of hostile obedience. They
wrote letters to one another almost every day for fifty years,
but there was much hypocrisy beneath the sweet and con-
siderate surface of that relationship, which as children we
did not comprehend. To us, Michigan was simply entranc-
ing. It smelled different, and Central Lake was so pretty
compared to Dobie, with mature hardwood trees and real
sidewalks and large wooden houses with generous porches.
It was a very small town, set in a lake-filled valley ringed
with hills, with cherry orchards, and stone farmhouses in
fields of corn, so there was an atmosphere of fecundity, of
cultural stability that was foreign to us. The interesting

relatives all seemed to admire Mom and be happy to see us. Our visit would be written up in the local paper, and the minister would single us out in church, where both sets of our grandparents had their own pew. I sang solos in church, and whenever I sang "Bless This House" I closed my eyes and thought of our own house in Dobie, especially in the climactic, soaring line "Bless the hearth ablazing there, with smoke ascending like a prayer..."

We learned to distinguish between what made us Botsfords and what came from our mother's Davis and Bowers lines. We always stayed with our maternal grandparents in a farmhouse at one end of a long gravel road. We were adored and spoiled by those grandparents; Grammy knew we loved her strawberry jam and cherry pie; Grampy let us do things like help him polish our white Sunday shoes and pick cherries from their small orchard. He had tools for Davy to admire and use.

But every Saturday morning we were made to walk down to the other end of the road to visit our paternal grandparents, who lived in a defiantly unmodern way in a tall wooden house with a gloomy front parlor and a woodstove in the kitchen and an ancient Dodge in the garage. Our father's parents were dour, eccentric, and even a little frightening. We were told that Grandpa Botsford was brilliant, but it was not something we could actually experience. He had a musty old butterfly collection in the attic, and he had memorized long passages of Shakespeare and the Bible; we knew these things, but they did not enable us to connect with him. Oddly, they had a television, and when we arrived at their house we were allowed to watch exotic American shows like *Big Top* and *The Three Stooges*. Grandma Botsford would make us a peculiar lunch, with ground beef and green peas mixed together on a biscuit, something that was not quite our idea of a hamburger, and then we were meant to sit outdoors and "visit." We loved their wild little garden and the fragrance of mock orange blossom and pinks, but we did not know how to talk to them, or they to us, except Davy, who could talk to Grandpa Botsford about his collection of tools and the rustic furniture that he made—chunky pine benches, rocking chairs, and a porch swing. I determined when it would be polite for us to leave.

We especially liked excursions to Mom's other relatives, on Torch Lake and Higgins Lake and in Mount Pleasant and Roscommon; even the names of the towns were beautiful to us. We loved our slightly older second cousins in Roscommon and Mount Pleasant—Butch and Judy and Nance and Joe—who mercilessly made fun of our accent but also took us to the miniature golf course and drive-in movies and taught us to water-ski. We emulated them desperately and always brought home to Dobie their way of speaking, for a time.

Mom escaped to those places because there she was not the meek and obedient daughter but an adult who laughed and shared risqué jokes and drank cocktails. Her parents were teetotalers, mostly because they were old-fashioned, almost innocent people who were born, lived their entire lives, and then were buried in one small town. Mom did not dare have a cocktail in her mother's house until very late in life. As small children, we did not yet understand the significance of what we felt as very different atmospheres.

WE WERE strictly discouraged from crying as children: *are you bleeding?* was the test Dad inflicted upon us. While Dad took seriously my recurring kidney infection (which required biweekly internal examinations, two lengthy stays at Sick Children's Hospital in Toronto, and finally a tonsillectomy), he had no patience for Davy's little hurts and worries. He called him a hypochondriac and sent him to summer camp to make a man of him. I suspect Dave grew up feeling unloved by Dad at least, if not Mom. But Dad did not express his feelings to any of us. Mom was the intervener, the interpreter, the one who took our case, for good or bad, to Dad. Mom told us what he was feeling: "Just wait till your dad gets home from the mine!" Or "Your father loves you *so* much," she would say. I believed that to be true, although I don't recall ever hearing him say so. Mom and Dad were affectionate with one another, almost symbiotic in their mutual reliance and love, but she was only at ease with us until we were teenagers and he not until we were adults.

42

As a teenager, the small "ornery" things about Davy caused Mom and Dad considerable anxiety, and over several years they threatened half-seriously to "send him to North Bay." (I am sitting on the landing at the top of the stairs, where I can't be seen from below. Mom and Dad are in the living room, in their chairs, having a drink, smoking, talking about Davy. Murmuring: *I'm at my wit's end, Jack*. Dad lowering his newspaper and peering over the top of his glasses: *Oh, my dear? What's he done now? He's just* impossible. *He was so rude to... sulked in his room all morning... and he will not...* I would strain my ears, dreading to hear the words *North Bay...*)

North Bay meant the mental hospital on the cusp of the hill on the northern outskirts of that town; the same hill that marked the beginning of the north also marked the frontier of insanity. No one ever suggested sending me or Sara to North Bay. But there was much rigor in our upbringing—rules, standards, disappointments, and cautiously meted-out approval. These things seemed to be about preparing us for the world; we knew from an early age that our destiny did not lie in Dobie. We were to be smart, tough, polite, sharp. Deferential to adults ("children are meant to be *seen* and not *heard*"), kind to animals and the elderly. The worst sin was stupidity. Our father would grimace and roll his eyes when we did not know something he thought we should—our times table, a date in history, the name of a bird or a tree. He was intolerant of slow or wrong answers: *Think, think, think!* he would hiss in exasperation, tapping his temple with a nicotined finger.

We were occasionally disciplined with the Green Stick, a supple, thin garden stake, which resided above the opening from the breakfast room to the kitchen, as a constant if infrequently realized threat. Spankings by our father took place in the furnace room. I don't remember being spanked often. I was not rebellious. My worst faults were getting

43

76

out of 100 on mechanical arithmetic tests, and I also ruined the finish on a carved walnut headboard in the guestroom by scratching it with a bobby pin. I would have said Davy got the most spankings, even as I am sure he was not an especially difficult child, just temperamental and very stubborn. In the inchoate way that things filter into children's minds, I understood that Davy made Mom and Dad mad.

But Sara thinks she got spanked the most, usually with the same hairbrush used to shape her shiny red ringlets, and once, when she was far too old, she was chased around the basement by Dad. She felt sorry for him and let him catch and spank her. Like Davy, Dad had a flashing temper. (I am in the upstairs bathroom, leaning out the window. Dad is on the back porch hitting Davy's dog Chief, who is cowering and whimpering; Dad is shouting at Davy because he is not training him properly. Davy is red-faced, shouting back at Dad and trying very hard not to cry.)

The curious thing was that even as teenagers, we could all see how similar Davy was to Dad, how they looked and spoke the same way, had deeply ingrained, echoing mannerisms. The main difference, then and always, was that Dad was at ease socially, gregarious, a teller of jokes, vain about his appearance, gracious with strangers and interested in their stories. Davy was silent; sometimes his shyness was oppressive, and he made strangers uncomfortable as he got older when he simply would not respond, make social small talk. He was not wild or rebellious, but he refused all his life to conform if it seemed someone was demanding that he do so. He had a furious temper, but once he was too old to wrestle with Sara, it was almost always directed at an object or himself: he might break a pool cue or smash a Ping-Pong ball or destroy something he was building if it was not coming together perfectly. Davy was a bad sport; he could not bear to lose at pool or Ping-Pong. (I am lying on a couch reading, in the basement, which became "the rec room" when we were teenagers. The walls are paneled now, the floor covered in felt carpet, and there is a stuffed swordfish on the wall, caught by Dad in Florida. There is a Ping-Pong table and Davy and Mom are playing. She is shouting with joy, leaping with surprising dexterity, almost dancing, and her aim is always unerring. Davy is getting quieter and quieter, his face red; he throws his paddle onto the table and retreats to the furnace room, slamming the door.)

When Dave was an adult and Dad retired, they finally recognized their common ground and found companionship in mining lore and the smallest details of engineering projects. They would sit side by side on a porch, each with a beer, and have long, muttered, fully absorbed technical conversations about problem solving underground and the state of international gold reserves. This camaraderie would make whichever Botsford women happened to be watching very happy.

We loved one another as children. But there was little sentiment in our house; our parents were not touchable, and they showed us no overt tenderness or physical affection, unless we were sick in bed. We were brought up to

45

infer tenderness. We occasionally saw that our father was blinking back tears. Our mother increasingly hid her eyes behind large sunglasses.

I remember Davy and Sara fighting a lot and me moderating or threatening to tell. These fights were knockdown wrestling matches; they hurt each other. Davy teased Sara relentlessly, called her "Zaa-Zaa," which she hated. They were both redheads with hot tempers and easily set each other alight with fury. Once Davy yanked a board from the floor of a treehouse and Sara fell out, tearing her hand on a nail. On another day he locked her out of the house after school. Sara and her friends once tied up one of Davy's friends to a tree and stuffed a sock in his mouth. Sara and Davy played a game they called hockey, throwing dishcloths at each other when they were supposed to be doing the dishes. Or they put two chairs together in the middle of the kitchen and pretended they were racing (with loud vocal effects) through the mountains.

I don't recall physical interaction with Davy; it was always the two of them. They were more together during the day, and their Dobie friends were a merged group of boys and girls over two grades, so they had adventures in the bush and schoolyard battles that I never had. I took to the role of the Goody-Two-Shoes older sister. My mother wrote me a letter, shortly after I married at 24, saying she was sorry that she had made me old and responsible before my time. But when I was a child it seemed perfectly natural to be above the fray, the one who knew the way to go, who organized and watched over Davy and Sara.

At night, Davy had his own bedroom, with a black bear-skin rug (the bear shot on the slimes) and his perfectly finished model ships and airplanes on display. As he got older he would rig up complicated electrical systems whereby an alarm clock would trigger a record player. Teddy Bear always sat on his neatly made bed.

Until late in my adolescence, Sara and I shared a bedroom. We had late-night routines, where she would try to sit on top of me in my bed, but I always got my knees up; she would beg me not to and I would agree but I always put my knees up at the last moment, and then we laughed until our parents heard us. Often we fell asleep holding hands between the twin beds.

Bless this door that it may prove
Ever open to joy and love.

FOR AS long as we lived in Dobie and Dad was the manager of Upper Canada Mine, the price of gold was fixed at $35 an ounce. The mine and employment in it were guaranteed, it seemed then, forever. The rhythms of work underground determined patterns of life on the surface. The mine whistle blew at noon each day, and the familiar rumble of daily underground blasts and the dreaded occasional rock bursts marked time for us. The mine bus that brought workers out from Kirkland Lake for every shift doubled as the school bus, which took us into Kirkland Lake for school after the sixth grade. But until then our frame of reference and the locus of our feelings and imagination was Dobie. My best friend,

47

Susan, moved away when I was ten, and I thought that was the end of the world. Davy's best friends, Lorne and Donald, never moved. Sara's best friends, Pat and Susan, moved in next door when she was ten. Davy and Sara were defined by these Dobie friendships until they left home for university.

But mingled with the coherence, the sweet sureness of the seasons that rolled over the landscape, the certainty of school and friendships, there were dark currents. These were cruel times. A Dobie friend, still living near Kirkland Lake, remembers going out to pick blueberries one summer afternoon and discovering the old black spaniel that belonged to Mr. and Mrs. Connors up the row from us on the hill, dead—tied to a tree and shot. Two boys who lived across the street from the Dobie school would be "beaten home" at lunchtime by their drunken father brandishing his belt. Houses burned down in the night. Children went in and out of foster care. There were Dobie families we referred to casually as "DIPs"—displaced persons. There were children in the Dobie school who smelled of neglect. These things we knew and took for granted.

Other things too were more subtly destructive, insidious over time. Environmental hazards were incidental, the stuff of daily life; PCBS were carried home from the power lines in swinging, open pails. In spring, a small tractor came and sprayed the lawns and the bush around the houses on the hill and on the streets of Dobie with DDT to kill the blackflies, and we ran after the tractor like the children of the Pied Piper and jumped and twirled in the billowing white clouds of poison. Although Dad was justly proud of the impeccable safety record of Upper Canada mine, almost every second family in Dobie sooner or later was afflicted by cancer or chronic disease. If you named everyone who lived there in one year, say, 1960, and asked what happened to them, there would be an exceptionally high incidence of early death, illness, suicide, misfortune, and alcoholism. My best friend's mother had M S. Sara's best friends' mother had Parkinson's disease. As adults, we would have cause to ponder this thicket of afflictions.

In our house this dark current took the form of jokes. One April Fool's Day my parents left a trail of red food coloring in the snow and told me that my beloved cat, Gray Boy, had been killed. One Christmas Eve, Dad put a glass of water on top of a broom handle up against the ceiling, gave the broomstick to Sara to hold, and then made the rest of us walk away. The joke was that she had no way of getting the glass down, and when it finally fell and broke, he made her clean it up. These "jokes" were signals to us that perhaps we should never feel fully secure, or unconditionally loved. We all had our version of feeling like the different or unwanted one—the dark side of being the oldest, the boy, the baby—thanks to our father's tendency to throw out the kind of thoughtless, jocular remarks about such things that children are haunted by. Mine surfaced every time we went out to Crystal Lake in summer, to the funny small mine cottage that was always ours to use. It had a fragrant outhouse, beside the woodpile at the end of a covered, wooden walkway, where I pondered his deliberately offensive phrase "nigger in the woodpile," which seemed to apply to me (or, somehow, the milkman?), as I was dark and

49

brown-eyed and my brother and sister were both blue-eyed redheads. Sara grew up believing she had been born under a cabbage leaf because by the time she was born, Dad wasn't taking so many pictures and that was the reason he gave her. Davy was mocked as a sissy.

People like our parents, who married after the war and settled down and quickly had children, felt in the immediate postwar years a brief sense of liberation and release. But in that bubble of illusory affluence and certainty, in the late '50s and early '60s in northern Ontario, there were deep traditions of silence in all classes and ethnic backgrounds. Secrecy was the dominant social code, ingrained during the war and abetted by a crisscrossing net of hierarchies based on religion, ethnicity, income, and job status; it was only in school that these barriers were erased, to be replaced by others, mainly scholastic and athletic aptitude. Many things, many forms of emotional or physical violence within families, were never discussed or admitted to or revealed in Kirkland Lake. Silence was the glue of our society. My family had secrets, things that remained unspoken. But it was only as an adult that I learned that other families had terrible secrets too and that the habits of emotional rigidity were common.

The violence I remember in our house as a child was verbal, and late at night, from around the time that I was eleven. Our parents would come home late from parties, arguing and drunk. Kirkland Lake was a hard-drinking town, in beer parlors and hotel bars and taverns, and at house parties, where my father and his friends mixed up gallons of a lethal mixture of brandy, rum, sherry, lemon juice, and soda water known as Boston Fishhouse Punch and served it ice-cold in small glasses that were never allowed to be empty. (I am lying in my bed, suddenly alert—the creak of tires in the snow, car doors slamming, stamping feet on the front porch, voices clashing in the vestibule, the hall, the living room. I pull the pillow over my ears and shut my eyes tight to drown out the sound of my pounding heart.)

It was when I was a teenager that Mom began to drink secretly. A pall fell on all of our adolescences. We became tense and wary, ashamed. Complicity encouraged a fierce sibling bonding, even as our natural tendencies at this age were to drift apart. Nothing changed, but everything changed.

In my midteens Dad's parents lived with us, causing disruption in routines and in our living space (I ended up in the basement for a while). My grandfather's senility, as we called it, was very hard on my mother; he would follow her incessantly, all day long from room to room, not knowing who she was, and he would try to enter her bedroom, which resulted in a lock on that door. She would retreat there in the early evening, with a gin and Tab. Ah yes, the gin and Tab.

None of us had a sanctioned or formally, happily recognized relationship until we left home. I had unrequited crushes on boys, but never a boyfriend, only hearty friendships. In high school, Davy tentatively, briefly loved a girl who was killed in a car accident. Sara remembers going to her funeral, but I never even met her. Sara had a long love affair, never approved by our parents. What were the barriers? In

Davy's case, shyness. We were all afraid to bring anyone home, in case Mom had been drinking. We were terrified of embarrassment or shame.

WHAT SURFACES: looking for gin bottles hidden in the bathroom, counting the Tab under the kitchen counter. Mom never drank pop or soft drinks (ginger ale was the only one permitted to us), so it was very odd that Tab (an early diet coke) became her cover of choice. Our searches were always done surreptitiously, as if they were the terrible thing, opening doors so quietly with a sharp intake of breath, running the water in the sink to cover the sound of rustling objects. She had sharp ears and unerring instincts. Usually finding nothing, and hoping to find nothing, but not relieved when nothing was found. Knowing something had been missed. We all did this, independent of one another, and not reporting to one another. Parallel furtive vigilance.

Her aqua-covered chair moved from house to house to house, but it always represented the same thing. Dad in his corner with the beer that smelled so wonderfully of hops (martinis came later); Mom in hers, with a glass of clear liquid (Tab was for upstairs, never officially a mix), sometimes hidden on the floor, at hand's reach, the ashtray slowly filling with half-smoked cigarettes, one lit from the last, long inches of ash, the scars over time that pocked the waxed wooden table, and latterly, the chair itself. Mom never drank and knitted at the same time. She knitted in the afternoon, fast and furious. She could and did knit in the dark, at the movies. She could knit and read at the same time. It was always a relief to come upon her knitting.

There is that wrenching theme in Eugene O'Neill's *Long Day's Journey into Night,* the father and sons gathered in the room downstairs, hearing the mother moving around overhead. Clocking, with increasing dread, the barely audible indications of addiction. That is how I recall this time: when she would retire and drink, and then get churned up by something and emerge belligerent, with a grating, flattened voice and eyes hard as buttons. "Go to bed, Louise," Dad would shout from in front of the television, when she would open the door to the basement and stand there, glaring or crying, swaying. And she would retreat, and come out again later, sometimes apologetic, sobbing, and he would tell her again to go to bed. What was she angry about? Why did we never know?

Some things: the early death of her younger brother, Jim, whom she had mothered from the age of 14; her virulent dislike of her own mother; her sense of uselessness, once we were past childhood. Self-loathing (she hated her body—she dressed and undressed inside her closet—the length of her arms, the color of her eyes) exacerbated by becoming an alcoholic, this secret that everyone knew, but that she could talk about with no one. For many years we did not use the word alcoholic when describing our mother. We allowed the phrase "nocturnal alcoholic" when pressed, or to one another. We may have said, our mother has a problem with alcohol sometimes.

What drove us wild was the Jekyll and Hyde nature of this furtive beast. There was the public, daytime, fun-loving and

53

immensely capable Mom, with whom each of us had sweet and goofy times. There were days or weeks of being "good" and then she would become this other person who cried, railed against life, stumbled and fell, was incoherent, and then the next day it would be as if nothing had happened.

I avoided the worst years by being absent. Davy expressed his disapproval by viciously imitating her behind her back. Sara lived with it as a teenager and under its shadow afterward because she was closest, geographically and emotionally. Dad's attitude in front of us was irritation at most and a fierce protectiveness if we dared to criticize. When I was 21, I wrote him a letter from university. I apologized for bothering him, "so busy with mine business." I said I spoke for Davy and Sara as well, about "the extent of Mother's drinking . . . I hate to call it what it must be . . . " I sent the letter "confidential/special delivery" to the mine and lived in terror that Mom would find it. The next time I was home Dad took me for a walk down to his vegetable garden, and said gently, "Your mother doesn't drink, but sometimes she's affected by what are called barbiturates."

When Dad died, in November 1991, that letter, carefully folded back into its envelope, was the only personal artifact in his dresser drawer, hidden under a box containing his war medals.

Why did he go on making martinis, night after night, year after year? Why could she sometimes hold her alcohol and at other times not at all? This went on, in varying degrees of awfulness, for thirty years. We would watch her, with despair and yes, contempt, sitting in her chair, with a cigarette in one limp hand and the drink, being sipped slowly, silently, and one slim, stockinged leg sliding slowly up and down the other, an almost sexual movement in a body otherwise still, the hated half-smile on her face, the slur and repetition overtaking her speech.

There was a game we played as children, in the basement of the Dobie house. The record player was plugged into an outlet that could be turned off with the light switch. We would put on "Ghost Riders in the Sky" and at a certain point in the chorus—"yippee yi yay, yippee yi"—right there, exactly, we would flip the wall switch and the music would go into a descending fall and the light would go off and there would be silence and darkness. We were in charge of this repetitive little drama in the basement. We could do and say absolutely nothing about the one in the bedroom upstairs.

IN THE late '50s, an entrepreneurial portrait painter traveled around northern Ontario, coming to middle-class houses to do formal portraits of the children, a deal that included identical, thickly gilded gesso and wood frames—$25, fitting extra. The three of us sat for this painter over three successive summers. It is impossible for me to say even now if these were good paintings; the likenesses were accurate, the backgrounds moody and atmospheric. The eyes were disconcerting, because when you entered the living room where all three portraits eventually hung, you were trapped by the gazes of all three of us hung on different walls, following you around the room.

My portrait was the first to be done. I wore a short-sleeved, pinkish-red blouse, very plain. Davy was next, and I suspect the artist talked my parents out of a shirt and tie; Davy wore a short-sleeved, collared, white polo shirt. Sara was painted in the beautiful pale turquoise silk dress that our parents brought back from Paris when they made their once-in-a-lifetime voyage in the *Homeric,* across the Atlantic.

When the artist came back to do Davy, my portrait was already hanging over the piano, where I looked at it every morning as I did my scales and arpeggios and Hanon exercises and Royal Conservatory pieces like "The Avalanche" and "Für Elise." I had decided my lips were too pale, too small, too *babyish.* When the painter was out of the room smoking a cigarette, I dipped the end of a toothpick into the color I preferred and made my lips a slick cherry-red. No one but me ever noticed this.

It was the end of childhood.

We still have our portraits. They traveled with Mom and Dad from Dobie to the mine manager's house at Macassa and then to North Carolina when they retired. When our parents died the portraits came to the summerhouse we three shared on Lake Simcoe in Ontario, where they again hung together on the living room walls, observing.

I brought the portraits of Davy and me up from my basement recently, dusted them off, and leaned them side by side against a wall. We look like conventional, middle-class children of the '50s—the children our parents hoped that we were, and to a considerable degree we truly were, before the rowdy onset of adolescence. We are caught in unlikely repose, with a half-smile on our lips, and my hands are neatly clasped in my lap. Davy is thin, his pale arms held awkwardly away from his body, his eyebrows pure white, his thick curly red hair cut short and slicked into a neatly parted, crisp cap.

The gesso on the frames is chipped and broken in places, the gilt worn, the paper backing is brittle. I tried to decipher the artist's signature—a scrawl in the same red as my lips—but I could not read it.

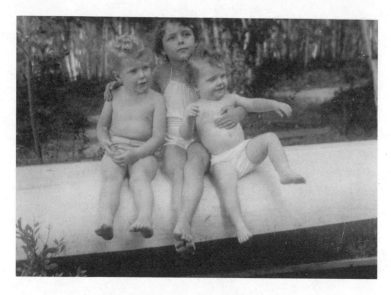

above: On the canoe at Crystal Lake

below: On a battlefield with Mom

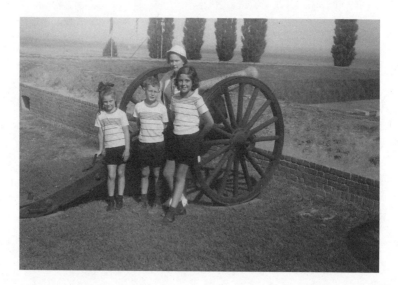

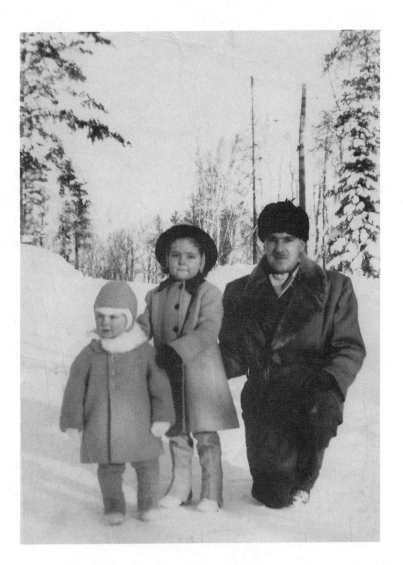

Davy and I with our father

PADDLE

TO THE

SEA

O UR way into Lake Beaverhouse on this day is via a boat-launching ramp on Howard's Lake, where we are to meet Dave's best friend, Lorne, with his motorboat and a rented outboard, both open aluminum craft with small motors. We are about five minutes late; Lorne, a lanky, serious man, is there with his boat already in the water. Jon says cheerfully that he will drive the other boat, though he has never driven a small outboard before. By eleven we are on the water, Lorne leading, Jon uncertain at first, until we move into the center of the stream. Their boat is too heavy, so Katherine moves into ours.

The air is quieter now. There is still a gray shield over the sun, and as we make our way into the long, easily flowing Misema River, the water is only slightly in motion. We are all remarkably at ease in these boats, on this water, watching for birds, observing and talking quietly. Our pace is measured. There is only one other boat on the water, a solitary native fisherman in a small outboard who seems to shadow us all day.

Our children are for the most part urban dwellers, living in Los Angeles and Vancouver, but they all have a deep instinct for the bush. For Jon and Katherine and Gideon, the landscape is almost familiar because it is like that near Temagami, two hours' drive to the south, where they had gone for several summers to the canoe-tripping camp, Wanapitei Wilderness Centre. Suki has never been up north, but she is a west coast hippie/sailor/traveler and she is instantly in tune with this place. Her questions—"what's a chip wagon? what's a butter tart?"—cause great incredulity and laughter. We all know that Suki is pregnant; Dave had also known this, ten days before he died. Quinn has only been to northern Ontario as an infant, but he finds his place because of the nature of the occasion and because he is with his family.

For Sara and me, approaching Lake Beaverhouse from Howard Lake is a backward journey, because as children we had always driven to the lake on the back road, out of Dobie, and put in at the southern end of the lake, near the old dam above the outflow into the Blanche River system. So the landmarks won't sing out in the proper, remembered sequence until the return journey.

Lorne knows these waters intimately. He and Dave were last here in 1994, when they came for a late-summer camping and fishing trip, in Lorne's old family canoe that could support a tiny motor. But they spent much of their boyhood together in this bush, and Lorne's family still has their cottage nearby on Crystal Lake, so his memory is not obscured by the layering of distances and intervening lives elsewhere in the world, as Sara's and mine are. He names the owners of the few small cottages—more like shanties, even toppled ruins—along the shoreline.

We move smoothly down a stretch of open river to the place where the lake itself begins, marked by the Beaverhouse First Nation's summer village. This point and this curving grassy bay, with small log houses strung in a necklace facing the water, are stamped in my memory. A white wooden church has stood there for more than seventy years, directly above the landing, and I know there is a graveyard behind the church. I have always wanted to visit that graveyard.

"Is it just an Indian burial ground?" I ask Lorne, over the small roar of the motor. He slows down, considers deliberately, in his way. "No, I don't think so," he says, "I think it's more of a graveyard for the whole lake. Remember old Alex, the trapper? I'm pretty sure he's in there."

I do remember Alex, a friend of our father's. A man who lived in a cabin out here all year round, who sometimes walked into Dobie and visited Dad at the mine. Or Dad would visit Alex, walking in on snowshoes in the winter, bringing him gifts, a turkey at Christmas, probably a bottle of whiskey.

Lorne points to the shoreline. "There are ancient portage routes running alongside these waters," he says, "down into the Blanche, or the White River, as they used to call it. Here it's now called by its Cree name, Misema. You know it

63

goes down eventually into the Ottawa River and then the St. Lawrence? You could go by canoe all the way to Montreal from here." Most of the paths would now be overgrown, but he remembers them as worn right into the rock.

This lake is still and black and very deep in places. Cliffs of granite laced with lichens rise straight up from the water's edge, the lake's history of highest water levels written well above this year's waterline. Scraggly jack pines and spruce sometimes miraculously have found toeholds, partway up the cliff, and they lean out over the water, seeking light. Here the rock is a pale gray streaked with green and a pink blush. Sara and I know that somewhere on the lake we will see a cliff the color of blood.

There is one very narrow, shallow channel, where large boulders litter the lakebed, scarcely visible in the flickering amber waters, where an occasional small fish shimmers. Lorne goes cautiously first; Jon follows. We cut and lift the motors and paddle through, aided by a slight tailwind and the surprisingly assertive current. I lean out over the small bow, scouting, pointing to boulders, remembering the last time I had done this with Dave, on the Coppermine River, eleven years earlier.

The channel deepens and we lower the motors and stow our paddles and sit back. This will be tricky when we come back against the current, we say.

FOR ABOUT fifteen years, Dave and I were not close. I went to university, then to England, where I married John, a New Zealander, and then to New Zealand. I never saw Dave play high school basketball, at which he was very good. I was not there when he got the mumps as a teenager—another debilitating illness, which went into his testicles. He went to university in northern Michigan (where Dad and his father and grandfather had also studied engineering), fell in love with an American girl named Kathy, with whom he moved to Vancouver Island. As John Botsford (no one in Campbell River except Kathy knew him as Dave), he worked as a mining engineer in an underground gold mine, as our father had also done. He lived for twenty years in Campbell River, which sits at the same latitude as Kirkland Lake, Ontario. He bought a house on the straits and had a canoe on his beach and the same breed of dog he had as a boy, yellow and black Labrador retrievers. He honed his skills as a woodworker, an exceptional downhill skier, and a road cyclist who did 100-kilometer bike trips ("centuries") every summer Sunday. In a very real way, Dave never left the north.

After Katherine's birth in New Zealand, we moved to Vancouver, where we saw Dave regularly if not frequently. Katherine created a bond, as both Dave and Kathy adored her and loved to have her visit, especially without John and me. She was a surrogate child for them, as were their dogs and cats. Kathy often said she never would have children because Dave would be a terrible father. John and I (and Sara when I told her) hated this comment and thought it cruel and not at all true. Our times with Dave and Kathy were amicable but a little strained, as we did not always warm to her. At times her vivacity was attractive and seemed a quality that Dave needed in a partner. Then she would appear abrasive and he would close in on himself. We knew Dave was eccentric, but she was also, in a completely opposite way, although fleetingly I thought that Dave sought in Kathy what Dad found in Mom. There were similar passive/aggressive tensions in their relationship.

After a decade in Vancouver, I felt restless and untested, disconnected from my own past and person and family. I craved the deep contentment and creative underpinning I associated with the north. The process of reconnecting took almost five years and culminated in a canoe trip down the Coppermine River with Dave.

I came east three summers in a row. The first summer I went to northern Michigan, to the town of Central Lake, where our parents grew up. I walked through a field one sultry afternoon, on land that had been my grandparents' farm and cherry orchard. Behind the house where the chicken house had stood, there was now just a faint outline of foundations and some scraps of chicken wire tangled in wild sweet peas and Queen Anne's lace. When our parents married in the garden of this house in 1946, Mom picked Queen Anne's lace out of the sweet grasses on the hillside and put them in Mason jars with food coloring to dye them pastel colors. Queen Anne's lace has always stood in my memory for our parents' wedding.

Now, as I stood in the field, the scent literally assailed me, wafting up from the sunny, sleepy field that was no more than a drift of knee-high grasses and flowers. I was conscious of the fragrance entering my nose and then my brain, and then I had a sharp sensation of memories awakened. It was like a truth serum.

The following summer, I spent a month on the southern fringe of Algonquin Park, as close as I could then get to northern Ontario, although somewhat south of the range I consider northern. North for our family has always begun on the ascent up the hill out of North Bay on Highway 11, the long, slow grind that peaks at the mental hospital. In an isolated cabin on Lake Kawagama, I was conscious again of emotions stirred by proximity to a certain scent or texture of the terrain. It had been almost twenty years since I'd spent time in this landscape, but I could feel knots of memory loosening. I spent hours on the lake alone in a canoe.

The cliff directly across from the cabin was one of those great faces of pink granite that give the landscape its bones. I paddled across to it one afternoon as quietly as possible, pulling the blade straight back in a long stroke, then flipping it sideways underwater and pulling it back through without lifting it so as not to make a splash, this maneuver remembered without effort by my body. As I pulled the canoe in close to the cliff, the temperature dropped; beneath the clear water I could see small fish and beaver debris. The cliff had the aggressive energy of an eruption in the earth's surface, frozen in place thousands of years ago. Ridges raked the rock at a forty-five degree angle to the water, and ledges thrust themselves out. The color changed with the light; there were sparkles of quartz outcrops. This was the rock of

67

my childhood. I have a visceral response to this rock whenever I see it. I want to lie naked, my bones pressed into it. I
want to breathe in the coolness of the stone.

At sunset I came home, hauled in the canoe. The water
was darkening fast; only the thin white birch and dead pine
leaning over the water were lit and could be seen as ruffled
reflections. The pink edges of the rock were briefly high-
lighted, but soon all would be gray and cool to look at, still
warm to the touch. The colours were softened and blurred
by dusk. I took off my clothes on the point and entered the
water.

At this hour there are two waters, the warm surface, a
foot or so deep, and a distinct chill meeting it from the bottom, a ledge of dark cold, below which the body hesitates to
go. To hang straight in this water, naked, face down, breasts
luminous, bobbing bubbles just below the surface, only
arms moving in a rhythmic finning motion, feet like limp
ghostly fish in the colder depths, is to risk connection with
the underworld. Or at least the past.

68   THE SUMMER of 1988, I persuaded Dave and Sara that we
should all go to Kirkland Lake for the first reunion of our
high school, the Kirkland Lake Collegiate and Vocational
Institute. Dave and I came from British Columbia; Sara,
from upper New York State. We stayed for a week in a dark
little cottage on Lake Sesiginika, the three of us together for
the first time since my wedding in London, England, in 1971.
Katherine and Jonathan were 12, and we had picked them

up at Camp Wanapitei near Temagami. Gideon was eight and Quinn a baby, not yet walking.

The cottage was a funny little place, typical of cottages built in the '30s and '40s, with a sloping roof, coarse screens, cracked linoleum on the kitchen floor, lumpy, slightly damp mattresses, and a smoky fireplace. Chipped thick dinnerware and a toaster that burned bread and lamps with crooked shades. It was like our old place on Crystal, we said, and somehow found room for three adults and four children and fell into the familiar routines of northern summer: blueberry pancakes for breakfast, canoe trips around the lake, swimming off a rickety raft.

Dave and Sara and I drove slowly through the town of Kirkland Lake and marveled at its shrunken, shabby face. When we were growing up, Kirkland Lake was like a medieval Tuscan town, with head frames instead of stone towers marking the seven gold mines. But now the main street, Government Road, was marked by poverty and the desperation that results in sudden fires gutting ill-kept buildings, leaving sad holes in the once-handsome façade along the sidewalk where we strutted as teenagers. This high school reunion was almost an act of defiance, where memory of prosperity and excitement and civic pride trumped the reality of a town left behind by its glittering history, for a few years in the '40s and '50s, as one of the most productive gold fields in the world.

Dave and I went underground at Macassa gold mine, where our father was manager for a few years before his

69

retirement, after Upper Canada shut down in the early '70s. We rode down in the cage with the current manager and a group of miners; I was collecting material for a radio documentary and I wanted Dave with me to ask questions I wouldn't know to ask. I was for one morning a mile beneath the earth's surface, in the small, black, hot pockets in the rock known as drifts, where Dave was completely at home, where he went every day as a mining engineer on Vancouver Island. He and the manager talked in the shorthand that men use when they both know exactly what they mean— about stopes and high-grade ore and rockbursts.

At night, the three of us went to the bars and drank raucously—beer with tequila chasers—with long-forgotten classmates whose faces and names slowly came into focus and then blurred again. We bought paper cones of hot, vinegary chips from the chip wagon on Duncan Road and went to the dances at the Belvedere Hall. During the day, we took the children out to Dobie. We made them pick blueberries on the hill behind our old house, just as we had done. We took pictures on the front porch, recreating the dynamics of the photos from the past—Sara acting like a brat, pouting and trying to escape the camera, Dave trying to yank her back into the photo by grabbing her T-shirt, me placid, hands folded neatly and smiling sunnily, as if nothing at all were out of the ordinary. Which was in fact the case.

At the end of the high school reunion, Dave and I drove back to Toronto together. We stopped at one of the roadside hamburger joints alongside Highway 11 and we took

70

our burgers and fries to a wooden picnic table under a tree, where we sat side by side looking into the bush, with our backs to the noisy stream of citybound vehicles.

"Kathy and I are almost divorced," said Dave, through a handful of chips.

"Really. When did this happen?"

"Oh . . . over the last three years, I guess. It's just a formality now."

"Oh," I said. "I'm sorry." He had never said a word about his divorce until then and I knew he would tell me no more about it. We got back in the car and continued our drive to Toronto.

They had broken up three summers before, in an exchange of handwritten letters. He kept the letters he received then, and no others. They are sad little letters, and they reveal, among other things, a man incapable of expressing love. A man either unwilling or unable to break out of his silence and isolation. In this way, Dave, who in so many ways seemed like our father, was the son of our mother, who also was very shy and had her deep abysses of misery. Dave would never have become an alcoholic. His addiction, if that is the right word, was to emotional inertia.

Our family did not talk about the things that mattered most to us. But in addition to the Botsford family reserve there was a deep, deep reticence in Dave. A pathological shyness, perhaps. Long before his body shut down, he was emotionally reclusive. An "inability to communicate" was noted regularly in his performance reports at work, and

71

obviously inhibited his advancement in his career. If he happened to shut down in front of strangers—by not speaking when spoken to—they might wonder if he was, in the word of the times, "retarded." The astringency in his emotional connections was matched by exceptional caution when it came to spending money. We used to tease Dad about being the slowest wallet in town, and Dave was even worse; he refused to play social games of gallantly picking up tabs. He was a good man, fair and utterly scrupulous, but he was not generous—although oddly, both Dad and Dave often gave thoughtful and beautiful gifts that the Botsford women treasured because we read them as expressions of unstated feelings.

After his divorce, Dave spent more time with me and my family in Vancouver. He came for birthdays and Christmas, and we went skiing together in the interior of B.C. One Easter weekend, he went with us to a lodge in northern B.C., where he and I spent a nostalgic afternoon exploring a mining ghost town. One summer day, he rebuilt the front steps of our house in Vancouver. He traveled to New Zealand with us one winter and meticulously reconstructed a kitchen door for my parents-in-law there. Dave shone when he had a project that required his skills.

In the spring of 1990, I decided on impulse to do a two-week canoe trip down the Coppermine River in the Arctic. The camp near Temagami, Ontario—the Wanapitei Wilderness Centre—that my daughter and Sara's sons attended over several summers also offered adult canoe trips, and I needed to satisfy my craving for the north. Also on impulse,

I asked Dave if he would come with me, and he said yes. The
trip would take us across the Arctic Circle and into the Arctic Ocean.

I have no idea why I thought, after more than twenty
years of leading very different lives, that Dave and I should
undertake a grueling two-week white-water canoeing expedition together. And I have no idea why he accepted the
invitation.

Remember *Paddle-to-the-Sea*? I said on the phone one
night as we made plans.

We'll paddle to the sea, we said in unison, laughing.
Maybe a little nervously.

WE HAD not paddled together for close to thirty years. But
there was no one else in the world with whom I would have
undertaken this adventure. On July 12, 1990, Dave and I
flew from Vancouver to Yellowknife to begin our Coppermine journey.

The first two days we spent in Yellowknife, sleeping on
the floor at Great Bear Aviation, across from the Wildcat
Café. Our pilot simply would not fly. It was our introduction
to the vagaries of planning travel in the far north. Weather
rules, or rather, pilots rule. Fog, rain, high winds prevailed
north of Yellowknife. The delay meant that we would have
to be taken farther downstream on the river when we
did leave, as our return to Yellowknife from the village of
Coppermine was not a movable date.

Dave and I had done no canoeing before the trip, and
as became obvious fairly quickly when we met Mark, our

73

guide from Wanapitei, we were old-school canoeists. We had to relearn our basic paddling technique on the dock in Yellowknife; our long stroke with straight arms, top arm high overhead, had been superseded since adolescent camp days by a stroke that kept the top hand no higher than chest level, and a leverlike motion with the paddle. Here we also got a glimmer of some of the special techniques that white water would demand, but we could not practice these until we were actually in fast-running water. We started to speak, though, about back ferrying and bracing and eddy turns and exits, consulting diagrams in books about canoeing.

Dave was experiencing shoulder and neck pain. He had had this condition for years, and he thought it was because of the two-hour bus ride he did twice daily to and from the mine where he worked, 80 kilometers from Campbell River. We decided he should get a cortisone shot, which amazingly was possible at short notice in Yellowknife. In retrospect, our delayed departure was a blessing, as he was advised not to undertake strenuous activity for forty-eight hours after the shot.

So we waited. We slept on the office floor of the air service and hung out at the Wildcat Café across the road. We circled around the act of bonding with our fellow travelers: our guide, Mark, a bright-eyed, quiet-spoken, skilled man in his early thirties, and a woman I will call Jane, some years older than me, from Boston, who had never been to the Arctic but had canoed in Maine and Quebec. Dave and Mark would share one tent, and Jane and I the other, so there would be immediate and unexpected intimacies with strangers. We were an odd group: four serious, intense individuals, each in our own way eccentric and accustomed to solitude and introspection. Dave was unusually at ease, but then we were in the north, his territory. It would take days of hard paddling to reveal our personalities and humors and frailties. We swapped minimal biographies, paddled a little around the bay, and contemplated the trip before us on the ordnance survey map.

The Coppermine River flows north and west, through the tundra north of Yellowknife, across the Arctic Circle, through the Coppermine Mountains and into Coronation Gulf and the Arctic Ocean. Its total length, from where it rises in Lac de Gras to the ocean, is about 800 kilometers; its contours and velocity range from placid, sandbanked lakes to rock-choked gorges where the water forms 2- and 3-meter standing waves. It was used for centuries for travel by Inuit and the Coppermine Indians, the Chipewyan, the Cree, before it was first traveled by Europeans in 1771, when the English explorer Samuel Hearne surveyed the Coppermine and became the first white person to stand on the shore of the Arctic Ocean. At Bloody Fall, the point where the river narrows and drops through a rocky canyon to the alluvial coastal plain, Hearne witnessed the massacre of a camping party of Inuit by the natives in his own party. In the summer of 1821, the explorer John Franklin also traveled down the Coppermine River and camped where Hearne had camped. His surgeon and naturalist John Richardson and the midshipman and artist Robert Hood wrote about the terrain, the wildlife, the people, and the travails of exploration. I carried photocopied pages from the journals of Hearne, Richardson, and Hood, which I would roll into my small purple dry bag to tuck up under the bow of the boat.

Since 1990, the Coppermine has become well known and busy as a white-water canoeing route and, I am told, there is an interpretive center at what is now called Bloody Falls. In the summer of 1990, we were the only travelers on the river.

DEPARTURE CAME abruptly and very early on the third morning. Our pilot, Bob Jensen, roused us with a plate of muffins his wife had baked and told us a brief window of better weather was expected to the north. Our gear was loaded into a battered Twin Beech 18, an ex-military plane with a Polish engine built in 1953, with 5,000 hours on it. The two yellow Mad River canoes were lashed on below the wings, resting on the pontoons. We were strapped in on hard narrow benches like paratroopers, and the plane took off like a pregnant duck.

From the air, the landscape was minimalist, dappled and bald in spots, sometimes very flat, then wooded, with myriad small lakes and rivers and streams. There was no obvious pattern to the waters; they were not joined by one river, and it seemed that a slight tip of the land put adjacent lakes (they looked like puddles from the air) into one watershed or the next one. We passed high over few signs of settlement: one native village, and a grand, sprawling compound belonging to Max Ward, a legendary pilot and owner of the maverick western airline Wardair. As the Coppermine River itself came into view, we could see it was at its southern end a complex series of small lakes imbedded in eskers. There were random patches of ice on the shorelines.

We were dropped at noon into the top end of a small lake, south of the mouth of the Hepburn River. Now it was just the four of us, our two canoes, and a caribou skull on the sandy beach. We loaded the boats—two tents, a small gas stove, an ax and a saw, Mark's guitar, our unwieldy personal knapsacks, heavy rubber splash covers for the canoes, cooking equipment, and the big, awkward wooden boxes called wanagans tightly packed with food, one in the center of each canoe—and entered the river: Dave and Mark in stern, Jane and I in bow, as it would be most days. At least three of us were nervous. Mark had never done the Coppermine, but he was a confident leader, with a compass, large-scale ordinance survey maps, and notes from previous Wanapitei trips down the river.

It was silent, except for a few birds and the sound of our paddles finding their rhythm. The water was clear at first, the riverbed rocky, and then the river became black as we passed into a deep channel propelled by the strong current. It was immediately obvious that the Coppermine was a chameleon. Dynamic. The anxiety of anticipation narrowed into concentration. The river had been impossible to visualize, certainly from home but even from Yellowknife, so I came to it with no picture in my mind. Being in the canoes, feeling the water running past and under the boat, brought the river into focus. It became real. It demanded our attention.

Dave and I felt immediately at home—with each other as paddlers and in the landscape, which looked and smelled like northern Ontario. There were many eskers—distinctive high sandy hills, regularly shaped, flat on top, descending to the river as pale banks, and then petering out as small beaches of soft sand. In this first part of the journey, we took for granted the scrawny, misshapen trees, mostly black spruce, which in a week or so, Dave pointed out, would vanish altogether. There would be no firewood then.

At the first rapids, Mark insisted that we beach the canoes, unload all the gear, and then get back into the boats to practice the essential paddling techniques—especially back ferrying and eddy turns, maneuvers that would allow us to slow in a current and choose and control a route through rapids. It was like learning dance steps.

The Mad River canoes, made of several laminated plastics, were both rugged and surprisingly supple on rocks. As we made our way downstream, we would occasionally leave behind a flash of yellow paint on the rocks, but the boats were exceptionally reliable and we became quite fond of them.

The feeling of paddling was quite awful at first, and it seemed unbelievable that we would start every day to do all over again what we had done all day the day before. It was hard work, more often than not into a head wind. The first day ended after a long, shallow set of rapids—a boulder fan, according to Mark—in a wide stretch of river. We set up camp on the west bank and had a glass of wine, and Mark made lasagna. After dinner Dave and Jane (in mild competition) caught several of the small, mild-tasting fish called grayling, which we hung complacently on a line in the water. We pitched our tents: Mark and Dave took the small A-frame; Jane's and mine was a small Eureka expedition tent with a tension-sprung dome and a porch, side pockets, a little window in the roof, and a net bag that hung down between us to hold precious things. It was odd to be climbing into this tiny, intimate space with a complete stranger at ten in the evening. She pulled a red silk balaclava over her face every night. I turned toward the outer wall of the tent. It was still light at eleven o'clock.

Overnight a large lake trout devoured the grayling and was in turn caught by Mark the next morning, with the tail of a grayling sticking out of its gullet. The rules of the river are disconcertingly simple.

OUR LIVES quickly took on the rhythm of the river. Dave (after twenty years of getting up at four to catch a bus to the mine) was almost always the first up every morning. He built a small fire and then took his spinner and rod down to the water. He was not a stylish fisherman, not overtly enamored of the sound of the whishing line or mesmerized by the sparkle of the water and the snap of his cast, and not given to a leisurely wander upstream like an English gentleman. Dave fished to eat, efficiently, doggedly. The business of breakfast—fish or oatmeal, pancakes or scrambled eggs—and striking the tents, packing the wanagans, loading the boats would take a couple of hours.

After paddling a while, a numbness of mind and muscle took over. We didn't switch sides very often, and I yielded to Dave's imperative, because he was usually in the stern and because he was much stronger than I, especially on his better, left side. This preference for one side reflected paddling habits stitched into the bones and had to do now with chronic pain in his neck and shoulder and later with a wrist that seemed to be sprained. We paddled for hours every day; what in life do we ever do for hours at a time, we wondered as we pulled, pulled, pulled . . .

We stopped several times each day, maybe for a brief snack and pee break or to scout rapids, and for lunch, which was a serious stop; we got out of the canoes and made sandwiches, rested, and wandered down the shore, maybe did a little fishing, usually Dave and Jane. Some days one of us, usually me, would swim in the icy waters, and afterward I would say how "gloriously happy" this made me. I felt clean and invigorated, and pain subsided.

When Dave and I were small, in a boat with our father, we were schooled in water lore. We learned to be silent and observant; *keep your eyes peeled,* we were ordered, paddling in the Chestnut canoe down at the lily-padded, marshy end of Crystal Lake or bobbing on the quieter stretches of the Blanche. Keep your eyes peeled, Dad would hiss as we slipped beneath the cliff on Beaverhouse in the big wooden motorboat or slid down the whispery grassy channel into the mysterious Sourdough Lake.

So on the Coppermine, as we paddled for hours on end, we kept our eyes peeled. We spent a lot of time staring into the water, trying to read it, trying to predict it, but we couldn't; we could only guess and then start to recognize potentially dangerous configurations of rock more easily. A pillow, for example—a shadowy rock veiled by a smooth sheet of water, some distance from a telltale curling piece of backwater—could be a subtle pattern to grasp from a moving boat and a challenge to plan a maneuver around. The morphology of the river—its bones and logic—was gradually revealed to us. When the water was flat and slow moving, we wore as little as we could while still protecting ourselves from the bugs and we left our piled gear casually vulnerable. For serious rapids, we donned raingear and tied everything down and the canoes were swaddled in splash covers, snapped on tighter than drum skins, from which we emerged, from the waist up, as if we were sitting in huge yellow hoop skirts.

We read the shoreline. The changes in the landscape were slight and gradual; a single feature, such as a low-lying esker, was really dramatic. It was the kind of place where you looked for and got pleasure from tiny little things—a sketch of tracks, a pile of dried scat, a scrap of lichen, or a single bird wheeling overhead. The banks, and even the rocky shores, were imbedded with miniature wildflowers, lots of dwarf willow and fireweed and bog violets. The lichens were intricate and elaborate, the thinnest skin of organism on exposed rock. We saw microcosmic family dramas: a pair of yellowleg sandpipers warning us from their nests, three moose, one young or female on the opposite bank, then a mother and calf, bounding up the hillside, silently, it seemed, as we couldn't hear them. We expect large animals to make a commensurate amount of noise, but moose and caribou, like elephants in Africa, often simply melt into their habitat. Small animals crept up around the fringes of our lunch spots and campsites, especially the funny little collared lemmings (we called them arctic fur dogs), with a beautiful gray coat and an elegant, erect posture, paws folded over their stomachs in anticipation of our crumbs.

After eight or ten hours on the river, we stopped, hungry, tired, in a jumble of emotions—exhilarated, irritable, or just battered, depending on how the paddling had been. In the evenings, Dave made the fire, Mark and I prepared food. Our meals were largely vegetarian except for the fish: grayling, trout, and farther downstream magnificent arctic char. In our big wooden wanagans, we carried a good supply of durable vegetables like cabbage, carrots, and onions. The flat wanagan lid became a cutting board. I became the salad maker. Jane murmured into her Dictaphone and consulted her Peterson's bird book and made notes about birds. Sometimes I read aloud from the photocopied pages of the historical journals as we camped on the precise points British explorers had two hundred years before us. We talked about what was the same and what was different.

It is only in the far north that we still experience a landscape unchanged since those first journeys, when Europeans gave their names and cartographic references to bodies of water and landmarks. It was much colder in July 1821, when John Franklin and John Richardson made this journey; just a week or so before our trip, massive, heavy ledges of ice still lined long sections of the river. Franklin's boats and native crew were burdened with guns, ammunition, and surveying instruments, which had to be offloaded and carried on the shore whenever the rapids looked as if they might prove dangerous. We carried no gun or ammunition and relied on double plastic garbage bags for sleeping bags and tents and small rubber dry sacks to protect valuables like cameras. For emergencies, we had with us one not quite legal flare. "Moschetoes very numerous," Richardson noted, alongside small hand-drawn maps and sketches of birds and lists in Latin of the same wildflowers and shrubs that we saw. But otherwise, the most significant difference between their trip and ours was the quantity of wildlife. Richardson wrote about herds of muskox roaming the shores and hills. Franklin's crew attempted to shoot every single muskox that they saw, as well as all the brown (grizzly) bears and reindeer, or caribou, and even birds like the little arctic terns. This land was no longer muskox territory. We would see one or two caribou or moose at a time and never a bear.

In the evenings it was so silent that from inside my tent I would hear a murmur of voices and think my companions were right outside when they were much lower on the bank. The wind traveled audibly across the hillside; you heard the wind and then almost a minute later you felt it. The first several days it was hot and the sun shone hard all day long and much of the night. The sun circled around the sky much higher than you would expect, and there was never deep darkness, even in the middle of the night—just a long, smoky twilight that modulated into dawn. This attenuated daylight was unsettling, and it perturbed our deepest rhythms. Robert Hood noted in his journal: "The first novelty that engages the attention in these northern latitudes, is the continuance of daylight throughout the twenty-four hours. It occasions a contention between the desires of the mind and of the body, which produces a certain degree of restlessness, till custom has established a change of habits." Even at midnight, if I stood and stretched outside the tent, unable to sleep, I would see just the beginnings of a sunset glimmering on the water. And my dreams were turbulent and relentless. I felt that I was climbing into a dream box every night. In Yellowknife, I dreamed of Polish cathedrals, though I had never been to Poland.

BUGS. ON the third morning it suddenly clouded over, and the bugs sounded like raindrops on the tent—big, frantic, insistent clouds of mosquitoes and herds of crawling blackflies. Dave slept in his pants but awoke every morning to find his legs gouged with bites, bites on top of bites. I wore knee-high socks, and long impenetrable Gore-Tex pants, but from the first nightfall I had a fresh, neat row of bloodied bites above the sock line. Jane and I were never without our bug hats outside the tent and constantly smearing ourselves with various substances—moisturizer, sunscreen, musk oil. I never knew what mixture was on my hands, which were swollen, puffed up, with bits of rash and many bites, so far no blisters, very dry on the inside. By the third day my $2.99 Canadian Tire bug hat was completely inadequate, too small in the head section, and the wires were poking out and tearing the mesh. I ignored Dave's snickers. Dave and Mark's bug defense was more primordial: they did not bathe, and they swaddled themselves in scarves and T-shirts, Arabian style, instead of wearing bug hats. Often we set out from shore in a panic, a frantic effort to get away, away from mosquitoes and blackflies; we believed that bugs don't follow you much once you get moving on a lake or river, but in the Arctic they did not know those rules and they hung in for miles at a time, only dissipating in a really strong wind or maybe finally in the middle of a very wide section of river, more a lake than a river. On a gray morning, we watched a large caribou with a big rack of antlers suddenly bound down to the water, shaking itself, also bothered by bugs, and then go galloping down the shore, running on sand and clumps of clay to the narrowest point, where it could swim across and come out of the water, up to a stand of trees, where it obviously regularly rubbed its antlers, then run down the opposite shore.

And birds... We came into a flat section of the river, with lots of open water and marshy shores and islands that barely surfaced. Sometimes we paddled the two canoes side by side, close enough to talk back and forth. Instead of heading to shore for a rest, we would sit midstream, passing a bag of dried fruit and nuts across the gunwales. We drank the clear river water, scooped up by Dave with his beautiful double-thickness stainless steel mug, which he carefully tied every morning with yellow nylon cord to the thwart of our boat. Jane (aided by the small binoculars she was constantly snatching up from chest to face) and I catalogued the birds so far: Whistling swans in groups, with distinctively straight necks and a kind of hooting bark. Arctic loons in flight and a spindly-legged phalarope skittering along the shore. Bay scoter, white-winged scoter, merganser, semipalmated plovers, a curlew or a whimbrel, bald eagles, maybe a hawk, or a small eagle, very mottled, and terns; we paddled past a low, sandy island covered in snowy-white terns, who saw Dave's and my canoe as a threat and flew up and dive-bombed us from behind, swooping low right over my head, stabbing the little triangular bow of the canoe with their beaks, unfazed by Dave's holler and paddle waving in the air.

But mostly we moved slowly down the river, knowing each day exactly how many kilometers we did that day. We were alert to the smallest changes in wind and current. Dave and I laughed often, but what about? We would talk, sometimes, and then go for long periods without saying a word. What did we talk about? What we saw and heard, mostly. About our traveling companions in the other boat. Dave and Mark shared the mutual wordless respect of men who knew and loved this kind of adventure. Our feelings about Jane were ambivalent; we struggled to like her.

I expected Dave as a mining engineer to know the geology of this landscape, and sometimes he did and sometimes he did not. We remembered how Dad always carried with him a small, Kissing Crane penknife with an ivory handle; he would stand for long minutes close to a rock face, unraveling the logic of its contours and strata. Then he would open the penknife and gently scratch the rock, then light a cigarette and ponder some more.

We too tried to put together the puzzle of the terrain we were passing through. The landforms seemed less settled here than on the west coast, where we lived—still showing signs of flux and the impact of weathering, perhaps because so much was clay and sand, and there was not much bedrock and the many eskers and drumlins and loess were just soft hills collapsing into the river. No stands of large trees lending a sense of immutability. The countryside was open, rolled back from the river, the spruce trees very sparse, the willows only waist-high; sometimes there was a smattering of driftwood stranded high on the shore by the ice. In some places the surfaces seemed raw, even tender; there were the porous rocks that broke so easily, and farther downstream we would see pieces of sandstone cliff fall into the river and watch slate plates as thin as paper breaking off. There were very few places of exposed bedrock.

Late one afternoon, we saw one, then two wolves, tracking us first from a low ridge and then along the east river bank. They bounded along, pacing us easily, and stopped near a large hole in sand, a den where they probably lived with cubs. They were beautiful, thickly furred, with very white heads and pale gray backs. When we camped that evening, after ten hours of paddling, on the north side of a small stream, the wolves camped on the south side close to their den, and we were aware of one another throughout the night, but not uneasy.

BY THIS time, the dynamics of personality were emerging. On the water the two canoes were like separate condos. Dave and I enjoyed one another's company. Sometimes I chattered, unable to resist wisecracks, which he always laughed at. In the other boat, Jane sang under her breath, sometimes aloud, from her impressive repertoire of show tunes. In the evenings it was almost impossible to be alone without wandering off into the bushes or down the shore, which was often impassable. I always tried to find a partly private bay for a brief, chilly swim. Jane and Dave took off in opposite directions to fish. One night in the first week, after a long, exhausting day of paddling we argued about our progress. Should we push harder? Would we make it to Coppermine for our flight? Should we travel one night between ten and midnight, when the wind was calmer, but the river was lively with animals and birds? Jane paced up and down the shore arms clasped behind her back like Patton and then took Mark aside for a consultation, in which she told him that Dave and I were weak; we could not be pushed. We in turn saw her as a lazy paddler, one who never took part in the chores, a moody person who seemed oblivious to the group ethos. Behind her back the three of us, sometimes giggling hysterically, referred to her as the General.

When we were just paddling, hour for hour, Dave and I clocked our physical state. A lot of this trip was about persevering, pushing through levels of pain. I was acutely aware of my physical limitations. Slow to start in the morning, feeling as if my blood were at a low temperature, almost subzero. And you don't just get up and go every day; you don't feel the way you expect to feel every morning. You hurt. You have been bitten. You have slept in a confined space, very close to someone you do not know at all and with whom you have oddly no connection at all. There are times when you are scared, but you don't get to process the fear, although your body does, by shaking all over, then and then again later. My body felt bruised internally. By mid-afternoon I felt my blood sugar level suddenly plummet and I would be weak, hungry. The first couple of nights, my body temperature dropped suddenly, noticeably.

Dave rarely talked about his constant and very specific pain. His shoulder and neck were not eased by the cortisone, and I did not know he had sprained his wrist until he casually mentioned it a day or so after it happened. However we felt separately, we paddled in perfect synchronicity.

When the river was fast it required our unwavering attention; when it was slow and wide, we watched the shores. The scenery slid past, subtle, slow to change. We watched the rock faces and clay banks for moving forms. The shortened trees made the judging of distance difficult. There were long, companionable gaps in our conversation. But also we were conscious of this silence as a way of becoming part of the country, leaving no trace of where

89

we had gone, maintaining the lowest profile possible for four white people in two yellow canoes.

There were few landmarks. Just before noon on the fourth day, we crossed the Arctic Circle (latitude 66' 33"). We took pictures against a flat, sandy, and unremarkable landscape and toasted the river gods with a ration of rum in Dave's mug. The next day we stopped to look at a hunters' cabin, an unwelcome window on how people had traveled more recently on this river. Dave and I became childlike explorers again; this cabin was just like the old camps, down the road from our house in Dobie, the two log cabins where miners were housed in the early days. We would spend hours in those buildings as small children, reconstructing lives and stories from the debris that we uncovered with heart-thudding excitement from under dirt and cobwebs and rubble. There were old lanterns and pots and pans and faded handwritten record books and shreds of old mattress inhabited by mice. The detritus here was more recent and less pleasing—piles of rusted cans riddled with bullet holes, and uncola bottles and mayonnaise jars, pieces of bedsprings and windows, an old stove.

Our silence in the boat was natural, companionable, and sometimes we shared observations just by pointing silently with a paddle: toward an island, where three deserted cygnets shivered, huddled together, later to a dead adult swan, floating in a bay. The river became a small lake, mirror-smooth under a pale gray sky, and we landed and climbed up to a small sod-and-log cabin built into the hill, facing the lake. We saw more caribou galloping along the shore, driven mad by bugs. Gyrfalcons hovered overhead. We camped at the mouth of a small stream.

At sunset Dave and Mark and I went for a hike up the hillside around ten in the evening. The walking was easy, exhilarating, as if we were giants wearing seven-league boots, the only people in the world, and we soon found ourselves bounding across a flat, grassy meadow high above the river. Mark, younger, faster, went even higher, to the very top of the ridge, where he saw arctic hare, horned larks, and the skull of a muskox. The skull was our first evidence of muskox, on a terrain that would have thundered with them a century or two ago. I unrolled the pages of Richardson's journal and read them to Dave as he broke up the embers of the fire; very close to this campsite, Franklin's party shot six muskox in a single evening. It was well after midnight and not even twilight when we went to our tents.

THE SIXTH day dawned cloudy; it was spitting rain. Our minds were wiped clear for an infamous stretch of the river known as the Rocky Defile. Even Franklin's party dreaded this gorge; it had been "the theme of discourse with the Indians for many days," according to Richardson's journal. We snapped the splash covers over the canoes, and Dave put on the same yellow rubber two-piece rain suit that our father used to wear underground. We reached the gorge in two hours and climbed up the right bank to scout the rapids.

The name Rocky Defile has nothing to do with defiance or even defiling; it was called a defile by Richardson, a term that came from the British military: a defile is a gorge that requires a marching army to go through in single file. Richardson and Franklin must also have spent some time on the plateau contemplating the waters below; Richardson imagined, looking at the contours of the surrounding hills, that there may once have been a long, narrow lake here, "whose superfluous waters were discharged by a magnificent cascade." But the river had ground down its bed by 1821, when it "struggle[d] through a narrow, gloomy channel which it has cut during the lapse of ages in the shelving foot of a hill."

It still looks exactly like that. On top of the cliff, we stood beside a monument to two canoeists, David and Carol Jones, who drowned in the churning waters below in August 1972. It was a brick, chimneylike plinth with a little etching of two people in a canoe on a granite plaque. Richardson and Franklin were able to go through in their canoes, but for us it was a "recommended" portage, according to Mark's notes.

This day, it looked safe to run. We discussed strategy: keep to the right (under the hill) all the way, said Mark; the biggest problem would be the large midstream pillow of shining water and the souse hole it covered, in which lurked an enormous jagged boulder. We made our way back down the cliff and into our canoes. Mark and Jane went first, and it was like watching a very good skier negotiate a slalom course; Mark was a skilled and strong canoeist.

Dave and I launched ourselves and started toward the cliff on the right. In the bow, I could not actually see the gorge, only ridges of standing waves, at least 2 meters high, looming over the boat, with curling foam that broke into my lap. We pushed through them, Dave shouting instructions from the stern between the gasps of breath that accompanied every stroke, every brace (a sharp *splat*ting move with the paddle). We found ourselves swept under the dark, cold shadow of the cliff on the right, because we could not hold the canoe on the correct angle with our imperfect back ferry technique. Then we were shot out by the current into midstream and lifted straight to the souse hole, which I did not see until we were right on top of it.

It is a paradox that water constantly running over a configuration of rocks presents an illusion of stasis. It seemed that time stopped and that we hovered there, on a shining curve of water just inches to the left of the boulder, until we were lifted up and over it by the river gods and tossed into the broken waters below. The rapids took almost an hour to scout, and less than three minutes to run.

We paddled weakly toward the shore and sat, heads buried in our hands, breathing hard, arms and legs shaking. We had taken in a lot of water, even with spray decks. Dave's mug became a bailer, giving us time to recover equanimity. It was not strength that got us through, but trust in each other. Unquestioning. Some would call it love, but that was not a word in our sibling vocabulary.

This trip had peeled away years of distance, silence, and our considerable differences in temperament and lifestyle. It had laid bare our profound respect and care for one another. Even though we would never articulate this, ever, we knew that we could absolutely depend on each other. From this point on, although we had no inkling of this at the time, our lives would become more and more intertwined, and one of us would need the other more and more.

After Rocky Defile, the landscape became more dramatic—magnificent red sedimentary rock, tilted, and then gray and crumbling slabs on the left bank, a long stretch undercut by river, like a series of decrepit castles, falling into the current. The river then divided into many shallow channels around low islands. A small glacier hung still on an outcrop above Stony Creek, what Richardson described as ice "out of reach" of the stream. We camped on the left shore below Stony Creek. It rained all night and the next morning was cold, cold, with rain and an icy wind.

I watched from the tent as Dave tried to nudge and blow a wet fire into life. He stood slightly stooped, pondering, looking exactly like Dad. What was he thinking about? The moment-by-moment strategy always. He was in a landscape where he was completely at home, able to do everything effortlessly—catch fish, build fires, portage, and do the hard paddling. I knew he was tired, in pain as we all were, but I also saw him as fiercely strong. In retrospect, it seems likely that he was battling with even larger vacuums of weakness than I knew or than he understood.

But we had become better paddlers. The river became shallow, choppy, the wind a relentless northerly laden with snow. The land tilted toward the coast, and the next several days were a kaleidoscope of rushing water, high cliffs stained red with shots of pure white quartz, and watchful wildlife—a worried pair of gyrfalcons, hovering over a nest with three chicks high on cliff, caribou loping along a sandstone plateau. Eight hours of paddling over a blur of significant rapids and ledges, soaked from the waist down, with huge pockets of water held in the spray skirts. Two more gyrfalcon nests on cliffs well-marked with droppings; the mothers cried at us and beat their wings slowly overhead as we were swept through. As we approached Escape Rapids, we fell in behind a flotilla of swans, drifting down the ledges. We had become one with the river.

When we stopped to rest we would lie flat on our backs some distance from one another and not speak, staring up into the sky. Or stroll along the river if we could; Mark found a chunk of native copper on the shale plates just above the rapids. Such scraps of rock and rumors of glittering minerals still fuel the persistent exploration of this territory.

Our second-to-last day took us to the portage above Bloody Falls. The paddling was rough and wet and cold; there was no sun, there were higher waves than we expected, and we had decided not to snap on the spray covers. Dave and I got distracted by birds (three red-throated loons and a peregrine falcon) and by green clay and sharply angled fault lines slashing the rock face. We got into some silly situations with high water and unseen boulders and lost our rhythm and the technique we thought we had mastered. I got the giggles and Dave got mad, slapping his paddle on the water and swearing. It was the only time during the trip when his formidable temper flared.

Bloody Falls was one of the few places on this journey that had a name and a story known to us beyond its coordinates on a map. Richardson called this site Massacre Rapids. Our campsite was exactly the same sheltered cove where the Dene in Samuel Hearne's party had ambushed and slaughtered the sleeping Inuit, that July night in 1771. In the early evening we climbed to the top of the hill behind the campsite, the hill on which the Dene had sat painted and camouflaged, in silence, until past midnight when they hurled themselves down the hillside. In 1821, when Franklin's party also camped here, the ground was covered with "rank grasses" and still "strewn with human skulls."

Our last night on the river was very cold. Falcons were keening somewhere on the cliff or on the plateau from where we had imagined we could see the ocean. The sun came close to setting, glittering hard silver on the rippling rapids on the lower fringes of the falls, where several swans floated. In my dream that night, I was in the back seat of a car that seemed to be very old, with leather seats, one of the only cars I remember from early childhood, the red Ford. It felt like it was early fall. When I turned and looked out the back window, there was a seal flying behind the car, and then it seemed to move into the back of the car, still flying, through the space where the window would have been. It hovered there with me, for some time. That's what the Inuit call a spirit dream, Jane said.

AS WE reluctantly emerged from the wilderness the next morning, the shock was physical. The river flattened and widened, first running smooth and deep and green, then broadening into the twisted ropes of shoal and tidal flats of a muddied estuary, so shallow in places that we poled our way through. No current left in the river at all.

The real world, to the extent that an Inuit village on the shores of the Arctic Ocean is a reality, encroached first in the shape of shacks on the riverbank, then the undersides of the hulls of big wooden fishing boats stranded high on the shore. Aluminum boats with small motors were carelessly beached. The riverbanks and yards were strewn with litter, and packs of dogs sat chained beside houses in the town. A large white cross atop the graceful spire of a pure white and pale blue church was an unexpected beacon. Its yard was enclosed with a perfect white picket fence, and on one side of the church there was a modest balcony for outdoor services.

The waves of the Arctic Ocean, here called the Coronation Gulf, resisted our approach briefly, and then let us pass along the shoreline of the village—two battered yellow canoes, four red-faced white people. We landed at the campground on the far side of town, beside the baseball diamond. As our canoe ground its way to a halt on the soft, gravelly beach, Dave lifted his paddle high over his head and then hurled it onto the shore.

Now there were trucks and ATVs and even a taxi, vehicles that go nowhere except between village and airport and dump, because there are no roads leading into or out of Coppermine. There is only the river. On the airport road there was a sign saying Welcome to Coppermine, but several years later the village reclaimed its Inuit name of Kugluktuk.

I saw myself a little later that day, in a mirror at Hugo's Café, the first time I had seen my face in a fortnight. (It had not occurred to me to bring a mirror on the trip.) It was indeed red, bitten, leathered, and my lips were cracked.

I lay on the grounds of the camping area with my hat over my face. I could faintly hear the sound of Inuit children playing games nearby and riding their bicycles up and down the beach, and swimming fully clothed in water where chunks of ice floated. The sound of children's voices would carry on into what elsewhere would be deep night, but here will be the longest, most lingering after-supper playtime in the world. I felt the tension of paddling—bracing, J-strokes, back ferries and eddy turns—ebb a little from my twitching shoulders, neck, and arms. An ice-tinged breeze moved the grass and small flowers and kept the bugs finally from deliciously bared feet and hands.

I thought I was lucky to have made this trip, in the company of my brother. I knew with every bone that I could not have done it with anyone but him. I was able to tell him so on the plane as we flew south. He said little, just grinned his little grin. The following Christmas, he gave me a stainless steel mug, just like his, with "Coppermine River 1990" engraved on it.

I knew also that this journey was not one that I could make again. Like life. That I could never go back was the distinction between this journey to a foreign place and many others.

The next day, we returned to our lives.

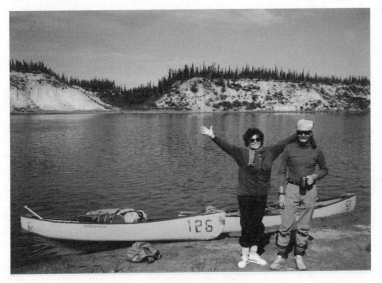

Dave and I crossing the Arctic Circle

3

THE

SUMMERHOUSE

YEARS

I T is a hot, hot day on Lake Beaverhouse. At high noon, when the wind brushes the clouds away from the sun, the heat is almost oppressive, but there is enough light movement of air, some mist, cloud, that we are never uncomfortable. The only wildlife visible on the water are loon families; a hawk occasionally tracks us from high above, and once, we startle a large gray heron in a small, shadowed bay, fishing. There are many beaver houses stacked up against the shoreline—large, surprisingly tidy piles of thousands of sticks, ends pointed by the chisel of the beavers' teeth, and ghostly, half-submerged trunks of birch and poplar, some with leaves still flickering underwater, catching the light. But we do not see or hear a single beaver all day.

We move slowly into the portion of the lake that is suddenly familiar. Odd details hurl from the deepest caves of our memories, where they have nestled undisturbed for decades. "Hey, Sara," I shout, "remember that place? That little cottage, over there on the island—"

"—and there on the shore," Sara interrupts me. "That's the point where we camped with Mom and Dad. Remember we had a fire, right there?"

"It was Labor Day weekend and I remember trying to catch a fish off that pink rock..."

"All five of us in that musty old army tent..."

The gray cliffs rise straight out of the black water, with sharp, angled edges and ancient small trees clinging in small seats of moss, the moss this year already yellowed and rusty from lack of rain. Some spruce, cedar, mostly jack pine, the occasional red or white pine. Off to one side, the channel into Sourdough Lake; now a large handsome cottage sits on the lip of that channel. Water lily field, pickerel weed, silence.

We go right down as far as the old dam at the end of the lake, beyond which we know are the remnants of the Upper Beaver Mine. This was where we had always put in with our parents in the big old boat. There was once a significant dam, we think, where now there is a gentle rapids. We have a discussion about where we should land. Lorne is a little anxious about beaching the boats, so he favors a bit of sandy shore. Sara is adamant about rock, for swimming. Jonathan wants to fish. It's an amicable sorting of familial priorities. Although we've spent most of our lives on opposite ends of the continent, we work together pretty well, as Dave and I had on the Coppermine and as we three had during our joint ownership of the summerhouse on Lake Simcoe.

We've already passed and noted the little island where Dave and Lorne had camped on their last trip, and this spot is where we end up. There's some flat shore for landing and a rocky point for swimming. A soft bank for sitting in the sun and a grove of large spruce trees lending shade. There is a ring of rocks on the little rise under the trees, ready for a fire if we could have one.

Lorne ties up his boat, walks up to the ring of rocks, and stands with his hands on his hips. "See right here?" he says. "Dave and I flattened a couple of logs and put them as benches, at right angles, close to these rocks." He kneels and pokes through old ashes with a stick. "You know one of the things about Dave and me? We could always come to a spot in the bush and make the perfect campsite without saying one word to each other."

Katherine and Jon take charge and start to prepare the lunch; they too are old Wanapitei hands, who did a fifty-day canoe trip together on the Coppermine and Hood rivers. Gideon is not feeling well, and he lies on the mossy hill, gazing skyward. Quinn is lively and inquisitive, probably nervous, taken in hand by Suki, especially after Katherine tears a leech from her foot after swimming. Leeches become Quinn's obsession for the afternoon.

I walk to the point. There is still a low rumble of thunder, far in the distance. I dive into the black water, through the spinning motes of light near the surface, into the colder depths.

OUR PARENTS retired to Hendersonville, North Carolina, to a tidy, sculpted enclave of rambling, bungalow-style houses with large lawns and gardens, filled with people like themselves. They were happy there; she joined the candy stripers hospital auxiliary, and he went to the Great Thinkers sessions at the public library and had his best vegetable garden ever. He finally grew the corn and melons he had dreamed about for years in northern Ontario, where he could grow almost anything except corn and melons. They went to theater and concerts in the area and made several good friends. I think she drank less. But she never gave it up entirely. When she visited us, there would be the pattern of days of even keel and easy good nature and then, almost inevitably, one bad night. Usually just one. The next morning, sweetness.

Mom loved to work as a volunteer at the hospital and thought, in her early seventies, about becoming a volunteer aide in the schools. But she became ill, resisting always going to a doctor, lying about how much she drank and smoked. Over several years, her health disintegrated, and she may have had a series of small strokes. Her right arm became stiff as a board, held tight to her body, and her nails curled into her hand. Her speech was affected. We, of course, speculated about what exactly she had: a form of dementia or Alzheimer's. But because she would not undergo extensive tests, her condition was only diagnosed broadly as a focal degenerative brain disease, with marked cerebral atrophy.

My informing memory of my mother was how she had cared for me at age eleven when I was bedridden. Now she would not allow me to care for her and instead maintained a devastating display of being "fine." Dad colluded in this.

The summer after Dave and I traveled down the Coppermine, I spent a week with my parents in the thick heat of
a North Carolina July. Mom's condition was shocking, but
they acted as if nothing had changed. She sat in her horrible chair and ate grapes almost methodically, dreamily,
looking at her left hand as it stretched out, maybe thinking
about the coming together of her fingers. She ate cinnamon
buns—three for breakfast, two after lunch—after fifty years
of never eating sweet things, probably a craving released by
not smoking and by drinking less. She demanded ice water,
tea, ice water, then tea, gin and water, one glass of iced red
wine, more ice water. She could barely speak, and her eyes
brimmed with shame and misery. She reluctantly allowed
me to take her by the hand, walk her into the bathroom, and
shower her, with a facecloth and soap as you would a baby.
I had never seen her unclothed. Her skin was creamy, soft.
She kept her back to me, panting, crying, and the words "I
am so embarrassed" made their way past her lips. But she
was cool and calm (*tank you, tank you*), for a while.

She had a red notebook in her desk drawer, full of painstakingly typed figures, crooked columns, some papers
upside down, but all the numbers correctly added. Over
and over and over, she gathered up the household bills and
checks and punched the keys of the calculator and the little
blue typewriter. She set the table for dinner: a scattering of
cutlery, mug tipped on top of spoon, fresh napkins under
bowls, all askew, but more or less as she wanted it still to be,
as it always had been in her immaculate and proper house.

Every night, Dad made her bed, turning down the sheets with army precision. He undressed her, tried to get her to take off her soiled, sticky shoes, but often she would not. "There, there," he would murmur, kissing her forehead, pulling up the strap of her clammy slip as he tucked her in. She would want to tell him something, and he would try to guess what she was saying. Since he was somewhat deaf, this was a nightmare charade to watch, as if the volume were both turned off and on high. When she sobbed and cried he got terribly upset; I don't know what she wants, he would say to me. Sometimes he lost patience and made small, mean jokes.

Often in the middle of the night, she would awaken from one of her nightmarish, shouting dreams and walk across the hall and crawl into his bed, curling in behind him, and they would sleep their troubled sleep together.

On my last day we packed a picnic and drove up the Blue Ridge Parkway, one of their favorite rituals. We found one of their special tables, overlooking distant rolling mountains. She walked with little padding steps, unsure of the terrain beneath her feet. She fell twice, once keeling over backwards, and I heard the sound of her head cracking on concrete. Her breath was panicky and shallow, her eyes wild. Her body like a welded unit, and her right arm rigid under lifeless flesh. She alternately glared and begged for help (*yes, peese...*). She was trapped in a box of horrible flesh. She had always loathed her body, and now in revenge it encased her. Sometimes, tears simply fell on her cheeks. We held hands tightly, while Dad smoked his cigarette.

In September, she was admitted to hospital after a fall. We were told by phone that the hospital would only release her to a nursing home. They intimated that Dad was abusing her; she was bruised from numerous falls as she stubbornly kept going up and down stairs, and he could not wash her or keep her clothes clean. I flew down from Ottawa, and Dad and I found a place called Cardinal Care and admitted her. It was an expensive place, superficially pastel and squeaky clean, but inexplicably where laundry was treated as a shared commodity, so people like my mother ended up in mismatched costumes they never would have worn by choice. For the first time in their forty-five years of marriage, Dad had done something against Mom's will.

On her first afternoon there, Mom and I walked slowly, arm in arm, on the grounds of Cardinal Care, down to a small pond where a pair of Canada geese paddled serenely. She was calm, and it was a dignified promenade. Somehow, she conveyed to me that the geese were her and Dad, and we laughed, and then she said quite clearly, crying, "I love him so much." I took her back to the room she now shared with a complete stranger.

That evening Dad and I drove in silence back to their house. I drove; he allowed me to put my hand over his, on the seat between us. He looked out the car window. "You'll notice, of course," he said, "the curves on these roads weren't properly engineered. You should be able to take a corner like this without making any adjustments to the steering wheel."

In mid-October, he had the first of two heart attacks (he drove himself to the hospital after visiting her in the nursing home and checked into emergency before the attack). They never saw one another again. The second heart attack killed him, on November 9, 1991. Dave was visiting them at the time, and Sara and I were soon there. Dave seemed to be in shock and sat for hours without moving at the breakfast table. I did practical things (banking and powers of attorney), and Sara took Mom to have her hair done and got her walking again. The retirement center found it easier to push people around in wheelchairs than to encourage them to walk.

I insisted that Mom see Dad before he was cremated; she resisted fiercely, shaking her head, saying no, no. But I asked the funeral home to dress him in his best dressing gown, with one of his beautiful stitched paisley ascots properly tied around his neck, and we took her there. She was wearing a red and white spotted blouse with a girlish neck bow and a gray skirt that were not hers. She was rigid with recalcitrance against me as we walked at a dreamlike pace to where Dad lay. We stopped beside the coffin. His head was thrown back in defiance, but his face was tranquil. I could feel tension and fear flowing out of Mom's body, and she was calm before grief overtook her.

She went to his funeral service in her own turquoise silk dress and walked in and out of the chapel. She came with us at sunset when we scattered his ashes on a rocky slope under Mount Pisgah, where rhododendrons would bloom in profusion come spring. We knew Dad would be amused by the idea of fertilizing the rhododendrons.

Nine days after Dad's death, Mom died in her sleep. The official cause of death was a heart attack. She had a very strong heart; I have no doubt that she willed herself to die. We did not have a second funeral service, as the first had celebrated their forty-five years together. On a foggy, rainy night we drove back up the mountain and scattered her ashes to mingle with his.

The following spring, Dave and Sara and I went to Florida for a holiday, to Sanibel Island. We paddled through mangrove swamps and birdwatched and looked into the sad eyes of manatees lurking under the piers. Sara and I walked on the beach at sunset and were a little puzzled when Dave would be too tired to walk with us. Several months later, the three of us impetuously bought the big, rambling, wooden green and white house north of Toronto that Sara had been renting for several previous summers.

WE CALLED it the summerhouse, though it was more or less winterized. It was part of a 75-year-old enclave on the eastern shore of Lake Simcoe known as Eastbourne. Here families still gather with ritual nostalgia and hilarity for carefully defined periods each summer; look after sunburnt babies, cranky four-year-olds, moody adolescents, and arthritic aunts; walk dogs to the store every morning before nine; sit on wooden docks staring at the passing boats; and play mediocre family golf and tennis and eat much, much later than they would in the city, especially on weekends, outside. The mothers and aunts and grandmothers are here all week, organizing tennis and swimming lessons for the children and enjoying the serenity of late mornings in shaded gardens before the husbands come up on Friday and rearrange the schedules slightly, but noticeably, over the weekend.

When we three bought the house in the spring of 1992, we imagined that we too would simply embrace this summer ritual. But our lives changed almost immediately, and the house became something else.

In early July, I arrived at Eastbourne from Ottawa in tandem with a small moving van holding all my furniture and books and belongings, intending to move into the house for a while. After twenty years, John and I were separating, reasonably amicably; our marriage had come to a standstill. That same day Dave arrived from out west for an extended summer vacation; the plan was for the whole family to do extensive repairs and renovations under his supervision. It was late afternoon when Dave and I got there, and before unloading we sat with a beer on a concrete bench under a huge Norway maple tree.

The house sprawled, even sagged in some lights, on a large lawn surrounded by cedars and maples, facing Lake Simcoe. It was green and white and had been since it was built in 1912 or 1916. We had the original architect's drawings, mounted on slightly curled blue cardboard. It was called the Scythe House, built for a family that made its money in awnings. The house once had green and white awnings on every porch and window; there were many, many porches and windows. Some of these awnings remained, ripped and frayed, coiled on rollers with rusted handles, but with their innermost layers still fresh green and white. There was one old wooden lawn chair covered in this original canvas. The house was a grander, if dilapidated, version of our house in Dobie, also white with green shutters and trim, set back on a lawn surrounded with birch and maple trees.

Tarnished brass lettering on a screen door said it was called Lone Birch Lodge, a reference to a single white birch that still leaned out over the water. But to old-timers in Eastbourne, it was still the Scrivener House, or the Tilley House, the names of its two previous owners, and it would not really become our house until we left or died, or unless we stayed for many years and our children married other children in the community. To us, this was the summerhouse.

Dave took a big swig of beer, watching a couple of golfers teeing up for the seventh hole, right beside our back fence. "I finally had that MRI," he said.

"You never told me you were having an MRI."

"I had it in May. I had to wait ten months for an appointment in Victoria."

"So..."

"I've got multiple sclerosis," he said. He showed no signs of emotion, and so I couldn't either (*are you bleeding?*). He said little more, except that he was relieved to know that his sense of feeling unwell was not imaginary.

"I've probably had it since I was in my twenties. I always used to wonder why I would get so tired climbing or hiking when other guys like Lorne didn't. Now I know."

From childhood, he had those odd little hurts, dismissed by Dad as mere hypochondria. Now certain episodes of fatigue or emotional paralysis as an adult seemed to make sense just because of those words, *multiple sclerosis*. The time in New Zealand when he shut himself into a bedroom for an entire day, the night of Sara's fortieth birthday when he simply refused to come downstairs so we could all go out for dinner, never offering a single word of explanation or apology. Because even he did not understand what was probably a sudden onset of debilitating overall weakness. Because he was terrified. I only thought, I need information. Information will give me the power to know what to do.

But we set this news aside and immediately started what we saw as a long process of restoration. The whole family worked under Dave's instruction that first glorious hot summer, washing, scraping, painting the entire exterior. We had the roof repaired. Dave—cheerful, relaxed, at home, seemingly indefatigable—climbed onto the screen porches at the back and painstakingly replaced hundreds of cedar shingles. He dismantled and repaired dozens of windows and set up an assembly line in the big porch off the kitchen for repainting them. He rented a compressor and blasted the old paint off, and then we all painted, for weeks it seemed. We gave the house storm windows for the upstairs porches and had the large trees pruned and made plans for the floors and fences.

Sara and I attempted to bring order to the gardens, where the yellow daises were taller than us and the lilacs so leggy they brushed the telephone wires. We tamed the most riotous corners of the bush and hedges. We worked from early morning until dusk and then had long dinners. One night, Dave requested a Mexican theme dinner, and Sara made guacamole and lethal margaritas, which we drank while playing croquet, and Dave danced around the kitchen with a big pan on his head, singing along with the Gypsy Kings.

We each took possession of a section of the upstairs. Sara, because she had found the house and had more children, had the master bedroom and porch. I had the next-largest room, also with a porch that became a study. Dave renovated a third room. By the end of the summer, we had made the house our own. We imagined staying for as long as it would take for it to become the Botsford House. Dave returned to Campbell River and Sara to the city. I lived there all winter, and then moved into a house in Toronto.

One day the following spring, I called the mine office on Vancouver Island to speak to Dave about financial matters. "Sorry, ma'am," said the switchboard operator, "Mr. Botsford no longer works here." I called him at home in Campbell River; his response was curt, monosyllabic, his voice soft. He had been "let go" the previous week, after twenty years as a senior mining engineer. We worked together with a lawyer on a brisk letter to the company president, pointing out the unfairness of this dismissal of a disabled person. He was immediately put on a provisional disability pension.

That spring, it was Dave who arrived at the summer house with all of his possessions, his sporty, low-slung Toyota Supra, his large collection of blues on CD, two large tool chests, the letters from the end of his marriage, and two childhood treasures: his teddy bear and his baseball glove. When he played catch with Sara's boys, we could see that his throw was weak, that he walked slowly and tired quickly. We started to clock the symptoms of multiple sclerosis.

Once Dave lived there permanently, our rituals evolved. We might all be there for Thanksgiving or Christmas. Over winter I came out from Toronto on weekends until Dave moved to the ground floor and sealed off the top floor to conserve energy. But come late May every year, when the lilacs and peonies were in bloom, we would start the preparations for summer.

THE HOUSE is quiet. Only the wooden floors creak. In the morning, light is filtered across little window panes, into rooms that smell of the sweetness of ageing pine, fir, and cedar, a scent verging exquisitely on mustiness but never quite reaching that point. This smell is one of the reasons we bought this house.

In the stretched and silent dawn, I become conscious of the modest hooting of the mourning doves that sit on the wire with frayed insulation hanging like Spanish moss. Later in the day, the cardinals, a pair named Louise and Jack—after our parents, who loved all birds but especially this official bird of their adoptive state—will shoot out of the cedar hedge when one of the cats saunters past and fly deep into the incoherent shrubbery leading to the back gate, where snowball trees and roses and untrimmed hydrangeas twist into a graceful overarching bramble. Rosehips and a scattering of red peony petals confuse the cats, and the cardinals seem to know this.

The mourning doves move into the cedar hedge. The filtering light becomes warmth, and the house begins to stir. This morning, there is still only Dave; Dobie, his yellow lab; my daughter's two old cats, Pansy and Willow; and me. Pansy sits on the well, where she can observe safely, with her back covered. Later she will climb the apple tree, enigmatic as the Cheshire Cat. Dobie sits on the roof of his kennel in his pen. Today is the day the family summer begins.

For the next month the house is bursting with people and animals. Sara, Gideon, and Quinn occupy the big bedroom and its porch. Jonathan and Katherine, both in their late teens, occasionally honor us with their supercool presence; they smoke cigarettes in the apartment over the garage and stand screaming on the dock in a thunderstorm and eat and drink voraciously and then blow back to the city, leaving a trail of our wet and dirtied sweaters and socks behind them. Emma the nanny has the ground floor bedroom and the adjoining porch. My sister's dogs, Sam the standard poodle and Andy the wheaten terrier, sleep in one of the side porches. Dobie sleeps outside, in his kennel beside the garage. But the sense of inside and outside domains is now defunct. Sam coolly usurps Dobie's alpha status. The screen on the back door is broken, so all the animals pass unfettered in and out, out and in. There is a crush of bowls and leashes and bags of dog food at the back door.

Days at the summer house are long, languid, and the house is big enough to embrace both our separate and entwining activities. Sometimes we have a boat, so the women pack vodka cocktails in a small cooler and cruise up the Black River with Sara on the bow in an orange swimsuit exchanging raunchy repartee with the golfers on the Briars course. We go swimming in the middle of the lake. Sara rollerblades on the road and plays golf. I bicycle in the early mornings or cool afternoons, down the dusty back roads, sometimes as far as the Sharon Temple, or to the graveyard at the end of Jackson's Point where Stephen Leacock and Mazo de la Roche reside. The first couple of years, Dave tinkers and putters with repairs to the house, replacing shingles, painting windows, fixing torn screens. He mows the lawn and spends long hours in his workshop in the cool basement and oversees the dogs.

For most of many days, women and children and dogs are on the dock, sunbathing, swimming, reading. Dave motors down on his AT V and walks carefully to a Muskoka chair. He kibitzes with the children and barks out fetching orders to Dobie, who crashes tirelessly in and out of the water. Gideon and Quinn form intense summer friendships with the other children of Eastbourne. There is a sweet return to the days of our childhood, when children could be outside after dark on their own, playing elaborate games like Capture the Flag on the little golf course behind the houses. Dave roars up and down the back road and around the perimeter of the golf course on his ATV, giving Dobie a good run twice a day. We adults have long, late candlelit dinners in the dining room, or we bring the tables out onto the lawn under the trees and fill Mason jars with dark yellow daisies and hydrangeas and invite guests and barbecue and drink margaritas and red wine and play croquet and charades and then go down to the dock to lie flat on our backs late at night looking for falling stars.

Suddenly, it is Sara's day of departure. After several hours the station wagon is fully loaded, the roof rack stuffed and rakishly tied down, the dogs bullied into the back, the boys in the back seat with boxes of toys stacked high between them, and Emma the nanny in the front seat under a musty brown mummy bag from the war. But Sam and Andy reek, and Sara fears she cannot take the stench for ten hours in the car (never mind the smells of unbrushed teeth and moldy toes and dirty clothes or the incessant fantasy chatter of Quinn and the prepubescent irritability of Gideon, unless he lapses into dreams of young Kate from down the road). She runs into the house and returns with a bottle of Old Spice aftershave, which she sprinkles generously on the dogs and generally into the already fetid air of the car on this steaming August morning.

And then the car lurches away, low to the ground like a cartoon car, everybody waving, goodbye, goodbye, the dogs excited, though they don't know why, except maybe Dobie, watching from the roof of his house in his kennel, who suddenly senses a major realignment of power.

There is silence. The cardinal named Jack sounds his single harsh note. Pansy appears, blinking and somewhat dusty, from under the porch.

Shall I make some blueberry pancakes, I ask. That would be nice, says Dave.

IT SEEMED that these halcyon days might go on forever. But by the summer of 1996, we knew this was not so.

. . .

July 12, 1996

How to chart the progress—no, the regression—of my brother, or the disease that my brother has become?

It is a sultry day; he lies back in his recliner on his porch, dozing. His feet are bare and reddish, sometimes purple, but he doesn't seem to care. He wears as always an old T-shirt, a pair of swimsuit shorts, and a baseball cap whenever he steps outside. The knobbly old cane I found in the garage a year ago never leaves his side.

The porch has become an extension of his bedroom, and this arrangement seems better for him than lying for hours on his bed, eating, watching his huge TV, reading. I do not see him doing much else. In the past two days, he has, in three separate forays outside, mowed the back lawn. To accomplish this chore he had to pump up the tire on the mower, probably each time. He walks Dobie religiously twice a day, Dave on his ATV, Dobie attached by a leash to the handle and pre-

118

*ceding the vehicle at a fast trot. Last evening I observed their
stately progress around the golf course, very carefully sticking to the perimeter, heading toward the underbrush when
Dave sensed that Dobie wanted to do his business.*

*His room and bathroom are lined with handles so he can
lift himself up and down. When he gets into the van, he hauls
his right side in by swinging on the steering wheel. Then he
puts both hands around his left leg to hoist it in, which sometimes takes several tries. His left leg is a stiffening, useless
appendage. He walks with exactly the jerky swinging hobble
that Jean Cheeseman had before she went to a walker and
then to a wheelchair. His left arm hangs most of the time,
and he does most things right-handed now even though he
is left-handed. I cannot tell how much use he actually has of
his left hand. Every single thing he does is hard.*

*The basement is a shambles right now, waterlogged saw-
dust and bits of wood and garbage cans full of refuse; he says
he is waiting for things to dry out to clean it up. I tell him he
should get someone in to help him. He seems not to hear me.*

· · ·

119

DAVE'S PROGRESS—like that of Bunyan's pilgrim, not one
of improvement—was marked by projects, year by year. In
winter '94 he built a plain pine cupboard and renovated his
upstairs bedroom. In winter '95 he made the cherry sideboard for the dining room and moved to the ground floor
and made the downstairs bathroom his own, with a shower
and a door directly into his bedroom. His woodworking
project of winter '96 was a kitchen counter for our friend

Frank's cottage on a lake in the Kawarthas. Frank brought measurements and pieces of old cherry, which Dave laminated. It was beautifully done, precisely right in its finished dimensions. He made the trip up to Frank's cottage to install it and managed the awkwardness of a long drive, a small boat, a wobbly dock, a rocky hillside without problems. It seemed that if he set himself a goal he could achieve it.

His decline was also marked by what was almost an annual shift in mobility and his strategies for dealing with these changes. In winter of '94 he got the snowmobile, which he used all winter, all over Lake Simcoe. In spring of '95 he became a man with a cane. In summer of '95, he bought the ATV, which became his life car around Eastbourne. I realized later that fall '95 marked the beginning of a time of huge activity and purchase, as if he had suddenly snapped out of a depression, an inertia; he was always unbearably slow to do things, in the eyes of everyone close to him. But there was a cool logic, an order, to his projects, only apparent in retrospect. Over the winter of '96, he sold his sporty car and bought a van, computer, television, chair—all big items—but he did not feel able to make these purchases until he belatedly received formal notification that he had been granted a long-term disability pension.

In fall '95 he experimented briefly with Meals on Wheels (depressing and quickly ended), saw an occupational therapist and a physiotherapist. The occupational therapist became for a while a watchdog, someone who could get him to make small changes and who helped him to research equipment. He acquired Naomi, a pleasant if bland young woman who once a week did his grocery shopping and cleaned for one hour.

His eating disintegrated; it became sugar based. A typical shopping list: red licorice twisters, a package of cinnamon buns, tortilla chips, chocolate-chip cookies, bananas, apples, cranberry or orange juice, coffee, bread, a frozen dinner, deli salads, a steak or some hamburger. He refused to spend more than fifty dollars a week. He went out once a week to rent videos and often stopped at the doughnut shop; one day I arrived unexpectedly around noon to find him on his bed with three doughnuts. I hated these moments; they reminded me of catching our mother sneaking drinks. He drank cartons of Bright's red wine one winter. He took a course of antibiotics, which he hoped would cure his long-term ulcer.

I made a desultory effort to improve his grocery list, going to the local supermarket, making a list of nutritious things. Sara tried to steer him toward protein when she was there, but as soon as she left, his next grocery list was right back into sugar. He insisted he needed quick energy, but he seemed to have no energy at all. I often saw him reading; I didn't often see him at his computer, but I know he spent time there, mastering the Internet and voice-activated software. His trips to the city became infrequent, and he could no longer stay with me; the stairs of my narrow Victorian house were impossible for him.

In the spring of '95, he made a trip to Vancouver on the train and flew back. The following winter he went to Halifax on the train; in Union Station he used a wheelchair

121

for the first time, but somehow this transition happened gracefully. He traveled with maps and the fattest books by Pierre Berton and Peter Newman, which he read slowly and thoroughly.

In February 1996, he allowed me to go with him to the MS clinic at St. Mike's in Toronto. I dropped him at the back door and parked the van. We went up the slow, dingy elevator to the fifth floor. It was a terribly long walk from the elevator down the hall to the clinic. (I have gotten so I instantly recognize the MS gait: body held rigid and slightly forward, a slight drag of one leg, a small twist and lurch.) He was a guinea pig at the clinic, we both thought, not a patient. A researcher came to take blood from us both for a study; another asked Dave to take part in a psychological study about inappropriate emotions, and, to my surprise, he agreed to do so. When asked about sudden outbursts of laughter or tears, he admitted to experiencing them. It seemed he could admit to vulnerability as part of a questionnaire, admit things he would never say directly to me. I had the feeling he was eager to be part of something, to be part of research, to reach out toward some kind of salvation.

But the doctor was almost cavalier in discussing possible remedies; none were for him, it seemed. He had chronic progressive MS, type A, we were told; less than 25 percent of MS sufferers are in that category, so most of the research and drug studies are done for those with the more common attack/remission pattern. Dave read to the doctor a list of drugs he had heard about; the doctor said oh, sure, maybe we could get that for you, call back in a few months. There was no analysis or diagnosis, no sense of connection with Dave as a real patient, a person. Just a file, a collection of observations over time. It seemed wrong to me that a disease could be called both chronic and progressive.

When we left, we walked past all the interns and researchers and doctors sitting companionably in the waiting room sharing a box of chocolates; it was Valentine's Day. Dave made his halting, proud progress silently past them. No one made eye contact with us.

.   .   .

Twice in the past three months, I have seen and been the direct object of his rage. I was scared, completely unnerved and deeply upset. Both times, the trigger was money, but we never got past the trigger because he erupted into swearing, screaming, roaring rage; I could not finish a sentence; he threw out completely irrational responses: he'd buy his own house, my goddamn lawyer knew nothing; fuck you, fuck you, fuck you. There was no space for exchange, just this side of his personality ripped open, revealing a red, bloody, screaming, contorted mass.

123

The last time, two days ago, he raised his cane as if to hit me, and afterward said he would only hit me if I hit him, but how could he even imagine that? I have often worried about his rage being directed toward Dobie, who is sometimes sneaky and mischievous and who knows Dave can't catch him; it's written all over the dog's face. I worry about why the

canes are broken. He goes berserk when Dobie runs away; he
cannot bear loss of authority over him, even when he knows
the dog's behavior is just that. And he loves Dobie as he has
always loved his dogs. But . . .

. . .

I CALLED Dave's ex-wife, Kathy, in Campbell River to ask
about his rages, and she was nonchalant, familiar with them;
did he ever get physical when they were married? I wanted
to know. Oh, no, she said. Fighting was an integral part of
their relationship and they both enjoyed it, but she got tired
of dealing with him.

In his desk drawer Dave had photos of him with Kathy
as a lusting young couple, when they married in Campbell
River in 1974. I found it hard to imagine the texture of their
life together; I only saw sparring, bickering—the small, picky
form of bickering. She would make lighthearted, sharp repartee out of his failings, which we were invited to laugh at
with her. His silences and emotional hollowness must have
infuriated her, athough they still had long, amicable conversations by phone.

As far as I know, Dave never dated or slept with another
woman after his divorce. He flirted obliquely with a certain
kind of woman, the kind with a sharp humor, an edge, the
kind who would take him on, get his subtle wit. Northern
women. I do not know about the impact of MS on libido.
He had one *Penthouse* magazine in his bedside table at the
summerhouse. But he was a shut-down person emotion-

ally, and ms drove him further into the solitude he already inhabited. His music was the blues: he had a high-quality sound system and hundreds of recordings of Buddy Guy, Stevie Ray Vaughan, Jeff Healey, Colin James, B.B. King. But he went to sleep for years, even before he was ill, to the plangent voice of k.d. lang.

I could see, briefly one night, as he shouted and I cried, that this interaction was a huge release for him, a display of vulnerability he shared with no one else. I did not want to be part of it.

I said things to him I should not have: don't take out your bitterness on me, I'm not responsible for it. And, you are mean, you are nasty. (He was mean in the sense of ungracious, churlish, stubborn, never offering to pay, having to be asked, never saying great meal or thanks or I appreciate. Not that I wanted him to be trapped by a sense of depending on me and so he had better be nice, not that huge sums of money were ever the issue. It was more a kind of civility that I hoped for and that he stubbornly would not give.) Even after the enormous fight, he would not give me money when I went out to shop for his groceries, but he was clearly happy for me to cook for him.

125

The inertia and pigheadedness made me cross, as did his slowness, sometimes a kind of deafness. I had to tell him things more than once, and he would forget he had told me things and repeat them over and over. I fleetingly recalled the rages of our father's father, who abruptly quit his job as the Antrim County surveyor at the age of 48, Dave's age. And the rages of our father's younger brother, Ward, which made him quit jobs and finally took the form of unarticulated roaring as he lay curled up in a crib in the locked ward of a nursing home, knowing nothing and nobody in his last years with Alzheimer's. This family history scared me; I'll bet it scared Dave too. There was a feature one day in the *Globe and Mail* called "Death Watch"; all the people in the story had MS, which finally led them to assisted suicide. They became trapped in their bodies. Dave and I both read the *Globe* every day, but we did not discuss this story.

In my bossy, interfering, unsympathetic way, I thought that Dave should push outward, not recede inward. That he should fight, not just wait to die or for a cure. That he should try things—if not radical treatments like bee sting therapy, then at least yoga or physiotherapy or massage. That he should think of every day as his last, or something closer to that than this passive lying in his chair, his bed. (Our family album is full of people in chairs: Grampy Davis died in his chair of a heart attack; we have many photos of the three of us fooling on a living room sofa, with Grandma Botsford in the background in the corner in her rocking chair. And Mom and her terrible, once-aqua, food-stained and cigarette-burned chair . . .)

But I couldn't make Dave do anything, and he simply looked the other way, read his paper, changed the channel, or talked to the dog when I suggested things.

By early August 1996, when I came back to the summer-house from a road and cycling trip to Nova Scotia and

Gaspé, it was very hot. Dave's mobility had decreased markedly. The weekend of Sara's birthday we had cocktails on the dock both nights. The first, he came down on his ATV to the grassy bank and then walked onto the dock on Sara's arm. I hated such moments: I was not useful, I got nervous, and I would make myself busy so as not to watch. On the return walk, I was behind them. Both of his legs were feeble and thin and white, his right leg now turned in, and his left leg was just a weight, and it seemed that everything from the waist down was fused. But he was more cheerful. The next night, he drove his ATV right down to the end of the dock, to save even that effort of the walk.

.   .   .

I think his slowness and repetition are a function of being too much alone, as if all of his social skills (which are few in any case and seldom turned on) have become rusty. Or is he just shutting everything down, the way Mom did in the year or so before her death?

I don't feel I have the skills to deal with this, and I am scared.

127

.   .   .

THAT AUTUMN was a time of increasing isolation, but he was in better temper and there were no rages. I spent one November Sunday there cooking and freezing the soups and stews of our childhood I knew he liked. I dreaded this exercise, because it took me straight back into the final year of our parents' lives, when I cooked batches of chili and beef and lamb stew and spaghetti sauces in Ottawa, where I then lived, froze them solid, filled two large coolers, and drove as fast as I could over two days to deliver them to Mom and Dad in North Carolina. Within a year of that trip, both parents were dead, and Dave and I were sitting at their breakfast table, eating lamb stew that I had frozen a year before. I associate a cooking binge with decline and death.

Dave sat in the kitchen for the entire time I was there, watching me cook, chatting. He graduated from canes to a very good walker. He bought a single hospital-like bed. He got the motorized recliner I had told him a year before would be the right one; in the meantime he had bought another, less expensive chair, but this new one really eased his life. I tried to accept, without comment, that he could not hear these things from me.

His life was a rigorous, slow ritual: up, breakfast (coffee, two or three sweet rolls, the paper), the first walk of Dobie on the ATV around ten. Rest, the Letterman show he taped for years, a pasta salad for lunch, computer work, second walk, maybe a shave. He went through old photographs, scanning them, making copies; he asked me to get frames. He depended absolutely on his routine and his aids, the tightening sphere in which he was comfortable. Some days he had great difficulty urinating, and disappeared for long periods into the bathroom, coming out, going straight back in again. I clocked these patterns and symptoms—I couldn't help it—but we did not discuss them.

When he first moved from Campbell River, he had out-fitted the basement with very good tools, and he drove around the area looking at cabinetwork and talked about woodworking as a means to earn money. The two large teak chests that he made for his collection of tools, some of which belonged to our grandfather Botsford, had pride of place. Once the renovations had ceased, he started with a small turned salad bowl for Quinn and cutting boards for Sara and me as Christmas presents and then moved on to bigger pieces over the next four years.

In October, he made a joke about selling his tools "before I cut off my hand." He then sold his electric drills and rotors and presses and power saws and with Lorne's help returned the basement to its pre-workshop state. The basement was empty now of his defining enterprise, swept, silent, a storage room again with echoes of his brief period of industry and creation here—the tiny black-and-white TV on a shelf, the funny upholstered stool tucked under the long workbench, the two huge teak chests closed and dusty, still filled with meticulously ordered tools. His two pieces of cabinetwork inhabited the dining room: the tall pine cupboard, his first piece, very simple, and the beauti-ful long cherry sideboard. It took him all of one winter to make the latter, and I saw him sometimes, pausing in the dining room to ponder his work, long fingers stroking the smooth contours of the cherry piece.

I became more and more his keeper; were we becoming closer? I could not tell. I was relieved when Lorne came to visit twice in the fall, and Dave really talked. He said then he would have liked to go to their 50-year anniversary at Big Doe Camp, but then said he probably would not have gone because he would not want people to see him "sick." He rarely expressed these feelings of self-consciousness. When he was alone he sighed and roared a lot, with every effort— of putting on a boot or buttoning a shirt or getting out of his chair. He was less vocal when someone was there.

Halfway through the summer, we realized he could not make the trip to New York State for Christmas at Sara's, so everyone came to the summerhouse. I made a list of things to be done before Sara and family arrived, and Katherine spent a day and night there and did chores, with Dave's advice; they had an easy strong relationship rooted in their early bonding on the west coast. He bought the tree and beer, had the septic tank cleaned. He was not grudging; his attitude to money had shifted somewhat. He paid me promptly and without making me feel I was dragging money from him. He lent Katherine his van over the weekend. It was with reluctance, however, that he turned the heat up in the house for the arrival of Sara, children, and dogs from New York.

On the Sunday before Christmas, we decorated the tree, had dinner in front of the fire. He had a moment when he could not get out of his chair. He refused help; he got angry; he pounded the chair. He finally allowed Sara to help, and then we rearranged the furniture so that his electric armchair could be brought back and forth between his room and the living room, and Katherine and Jon were helpful and strong.

Pat the occupational therapist came with plastic stools for him to use to get in and out of his van. Dave described to her and me how he did things: he put the walker on the back of the ATV, drove to the garage and opened the door, opened the car driver's door, walked the walker around to the passenger side and put it in, then edged back along the van to his door and got in. Repeating the whole process at his destination, twice, then again when he got home.

We talked about places he might move to, and he said he would start researching the possibilities in January. Pat had already told me she knew she had to give him a huge amount of time to consider everything. She liked his sharp sense of humor. He was almost lighthearted with her—clear, open, in a way that Sara and I seldom saw. He said that when he got to the stage where he couldn't get out of bed or shower by himself there would be no point in staying at the summerhouse. He really would like a place in the country, he said, where he could still have Dobie. As he spoke, I felt he was confronting a likelihood he had not really considered much. Or maybe he thought about it every night when he woke up and could not get back to sleep, but this exchange was the first time we had what might be thought of as a caregiving, planning conversation. (Quinn, who was only nine, said to Sara, "Dave should be in a place with five or six people like him, so they can talk together. And the apartments should be set up so there isn't stuff in the way and not be very big so it is easy to get around. And there could be someone who comes to help them when they need that." There were few such places.)

131

The next day, I cried all the way to Newmarket. I went to every single shoe store in the Upper Canada Mall looking for snowboots "for my brother. He's disabled; he needs something low, with a zipper or Velcro, no laces." There was no such boot. There was a plethora of options for people who did not need choice, but nothing for someone who required something that was exactly right.

Christmas morning was a perfect wintry day, a thick blanket of fresh snow on the lawn and trees, and fat flakes that flew on and off all day long. I gave Sara a wine bottle stopper in her stocking. Dave said, "That's for when the house is burning down and you have to get out quickly with your open bottle of wine." This became a classic family joke, like Dave's other Christmas joke that we recall every year: when he was about Quinn's age, he looked at some antiqued end tables our father had bought our mother and said, "Those look like something Joseph made on Christmas Eve."

We had a great day, with good presents and late breakfast and a long family walk on the snow-covered golf course, with the dogs and cameras and much suiting up ahead of time. Dave was on the ATV roaring out ahead, the only chance he had to feel speed, wind, acceleration, exhilaration. The only time he was not visibly disabled and immobile and different. He was wearing his Whistler ski cap and an old red ski jacket, and I pictured him on his skis, the long, whipping ripple of his flight down a mountain. I wondered if this was how he appeared in his dreams.

Before the end of the week, I drove to Newmarket twice in one day, trying again fruitlessly to get boots but coming back with a pair of backless slippers, a new phone. He was gracious. And then it was the end of the week and we cleaned up everything, took down the tree and the mantle decorations, and stripped the beds and sealed the upstairs heating vents and placed the Styrofoam back over the stairwell and went away, with our children, dogs, presents, our presence. And the house was silent, dark, cold, and Dave was alone with Dobie.

IT WAS a hard winter. The snow was swept high in drifts against the exterior walls of the house, where it was met by huge icicles crawling downward. A fox often glowered at the house from the shadow of the ice-laden trees that fringed the garden. One bitterly cold day in January, I drove out from the city because Dave reluctantly called me. His snowmobile battery had died, and the sewage pipes in the house were frozen, and Dobie was running around in circles inside the house. I thawed the pipes with a heater under the floor and poured hot water down the toilet and charged up the battery and took Dobie out for a walk.

Within an hour of my leaving to drive back to Toronto, Dave took Dobie for a run alongside his snowmobile and fell on his return as he dismounted, right beside the house. For fifteen minutes, he struggled, face down in the snow, and I know that means he was swearing and keening, the high, thin sound he had started to make when he was thwarted trying to do something physical, a sound that contorted his face and throat and drew ebbing energy away from the task he was trying to complete. It was already dark; Dobie was dashing to and fro, and finally he ran down the path, along the back road to the house of his dog friend, Keswick, next door, possibly knowing that he might get help for Dave this way. Dave crawled on his stomach up the two steps, across the threshold of the little porch, and at least partway through the door into the house. This trek took him forty-five minutes, and it was how Peter, the next-door neighbor, found him. The next day, he got stuck on the golf course on his snowmobile and telephoned Peter to call someone to pull him out. Within days, he sold his snowmobile and got a MedAlert bracelet and an electric wheelchair and told me we should start looking for a place for him to live. I spent the next two months in overdrive, making applications and appointments and badgering managers on the phone and making snap decisions.

By the end of April, he had moved into Windward Co-operative, beside Lake Ontario, in Toronto, a small-scale, pleasant, wheelchair-accessible building with both able and disabled residents and lots of people with dogs and easy access to the walks along the lake, and only a five-minute drive from my house. On good days, he could even motor up to my house on his wheelchair. We had a wheelchair lift installed in his van and bought a set of portable, metal ramps to use at my house and at the summerhouse. He got a floor-to-ceiling pole to put beside his bed, to help him get in and out of bed, and a bath chair and a toilet seat. The paraphernalia of disability began to accumulate. But the electric wheelchair was liberating, although once he began using it, he never walked again. He began, gradually at first, to rely on the services of Participation, an assisted-care unit with offices in his building.

We developed rituals for this new proximity. It was easy for me to come on my bike to cook a meal, and we would go for long walks along the lakefront. He looped Dobie's leash through the arm of his wheelchair, and Dobie trotted and I either walked briskly or sometimes rode my bike. It was a beautiful walk, past the yacht basins and the old warship *Haida* tethered near the walkway, past the Ontario Pavilion complex and the rowing clubs. On fine days, we would go as far as we could, past the graceful, spidery arch of the Humber Bridge. We would stop for French fries or an ice cream and sit facing the water, watching the sunset or fireworks or a boat race. Some days we took a picnic. When I was not there, he and Dobie did a version of this waterfront walk every single day, often more than once. In the summer, he moved out to the summerhouse and Sara and the boys came and we resumed the lives of summer people.

That autumn, the light shifted again. Dave and I went out to the summerhouse one afternoon to shut off the water and close down the house for winter, as we knew we would not be back again until the following spring. He disappeared into his bathroom for more than an hour. He refused my neutrally voiced offers of help and finally slowly emerged, painstakingly maneuvering his wheelchair down the metal ramps onto the lawn. There were feces smeared on his ankles and feet.

"Would you like me to bathe your feet before we head home?" I asked. He nodded, so I filled an enamel basin with warm water and soap and sat on the grass and washed him carefully with an old hand towel.

"This might be the last time I see Lone Birch Lodge," he said. I did not know how to reply. We turned and watched the late-afternoon sun set ablaze the red and yellow canopy of trees across the golf course.

A month later his body seized up one afternoon and he went into shock, head lolling, right side of his face shut down, unable to hold his eyelid open, sitting in the wheelchair with his arms crossed, completely paralyzed. We had our first experience of ambulances and emergency room chaos; at St. Mike's, six people were ahead of Dave waiting for a bed, so after six hours he was moved to Toronto Western. He had a high temperature, could not move his left arm away from his body, and felt acute pain in his left arm when his right arm was touched. He appeared to recover and was desperate to go home, but the next afternoon he went into spasms, shaking all over, crying out in pain. Desultory nurses took their time in getting to him, were irritated when he was unable to close his mouth around a thermometer, and snapped at him for hollering involuntarily during the night. I sat beside his bed for several hours; he was shuddering, in a blue hospital gown that was falling off one shoulder. His body was big and white, and his hands kept reaching out, clutching at his right thigh. His legs were immobile—one knee out, feet crossed in an involuntary crucifixion position. He was oblivious to a tray of rubbery meatballs, but finally he asked me to feed him a few bites, which I did, never having fed him before.

This interlude marked the emergence of the rottweiler persona that Sara and I would assume from now on whenever Dave's condition got worse and we had to engage with the medical establishment. These interactions required unexpected, aggressive vigilance. In the emergency room at St. Mike's, his lung X-rays were mixed up with those of another patient. At Toronto Western, important information was repeatedly not written on his chart. The nurses neglected to catheterize him, and he was incontinent in the night and yelling; was he in pain, the irritated nurse would ask, and he would say no, he just wanted to be sure there was someone there. I found myself wondering if there was a person here I didn't know, someone who was hiding terror and long-term incontinence from me, whose condition was far worse than I knew. Was there a huge subterfuge, a small subterfuge? Protect, deny; sometimes when I looked at Dave, I saw Mom. When asked by a doctor he said, I've been just fine the last few days, no, no problems, and I said, but don't you remember, Saturday I had to come and pick you up off the floor, and again on Tuesday I had to come? Denying or forgetting . . .

But later he said, "I woke up two or three times last night and found myself shouting. I was pretty embarrassed." He grimaced.

"Oh, oh," I said, jokingly. "Now you're turning into Mom. Remember those horrible nightmares she used to have, shouting really loud?"

He half winced, half laughed, and his hands tugged at the damp sheet as he tried to shift his weight. I wedged a

137

pillow between his ankles. "Thank you," he said. A pause. "And not only that, I was soaking wet. Apparently I'd pissed myself."

I took this revelation as a sign that he was not lying to me.

A nurse or nurse practitioner (nobody wears a uniform anymore) came toward him with purpose and a couple of towels and a fresh gown.

He said quietly, "You might want to leave the room while I'm cleaned up."

I came back later while he dozed, his limbs sometimes jumping a little, twitching, his body incapable of stretching or curling or rolling over. I pulled the sheet over him and sat in the hard chair. I recalled a conversation with a friend about how the body is not the person. The body is not the person to the person inside the body.

What barriers there had been between Dave and me were broken down by his being in hospital, my feeding him, talking about incontinence, seeing him with a ratty towel between his legs, patting his head, stroking his hair, giving the kind of compassion that normally would not be easy for me to display to him or for him to receive from me. Because he was trapped, in the hospital, our relationship became more intimate.

But there were two Daves. One was impassive and stalwart, apparently impervious to pain and discomfort. That one who said "fine" whenever you asked him how he was, despite compelling evidence to the contrary. The other was the man whose feet were bloodied from bashing into the bathroom wall with his wheelchair. Whose face twisted with frustration, neck muscles distended, mouth open, with the effort of completing some deceptively small movement. Who, behind a closed door, broke into a soft keening, heart-rending waves of high, sweet, almost falsetto cries, like the bleating of a trapped bird. At times the bleating became a full-throated roaring, the sound of a primate wounded, in terrible pain. But if you knocked on the door, or called out to him in the middle of this aria—Dave, are you okay? Dave, can I help?—he always replied without hesitation in the calm, measured tones of someone reading a book on the toilet—no, thank you, I am fine. And there would be a small silence.

I too was immobilized, sitting in a chair at the end of his bed, watching the light drain from the western sky over the city, closing out the whispered argument the man in the next bed was having with his wife. Thinking, now is the time when you want to be a knitter.

THE FOLLOWING summer, Dave did come back to the summerhouse, for almost two months. It was one of our best summers. Jon introduced us to Suki and proposed to her. We celebrated on the dock, sitting in a circle and passing the bottle of champagne like a talking stick. We all proffered our opinions on the wedding and on the future of the summerhouse, which was becoming increasingly difficult for the three of us to manage.

On the last day of August, Jon and Suki were married, in a ceremony at sunset on the dock. All of our complicated family was there. It was a perfect late-summer evening, the air still and cool, the light like liquid amber. We had dinner on the lawn and danced outside until four in the morning on a rented dance floor lit with torches.

The next day, everyone vanished to the corners of the continent and I supervised the separation of possessions into three piles to be shipped or stored. We had sold the summerhouse.

Dave and I went to California for Christmas. He was immobile on the plane for five hours and ill prepared for the flight; on arrival in Los Angeles, he wheeled himself into a washroom and did not, would not, emerge, for two hours. (Before the return journey, he prepared himself; we kept learning new things, unexpectedly.) In Sara's small house in Studio City, he struggled at first with the new environment, crashing into walls, panicking because he could not see at first how he could use the toilet; the sink was on the left, so he had trouble turning on the tap, and he couldn't turn his chair, so he had to back out: all the things you don't think about until they happen. His bed was soft, and when he stiffened up in the night, he could not get up and he groaned and keened, and I was in the room next door and got up most nights to help him get up. He always had to get up.

But we rented a wonderful, luxurious van, a sleek silver elephant, that seemed to kneel, hydraulically, before folding down its built-in ramp. And the air was soft and not too hot, so he went outdoors in shorts and bare feet, up and down the road, to the little park or over to the main street for coffee; these small pieces of mobility were exhilarating. The three of us roared down the coast to San Diego, where the motel had a high bed and a wheel-in shower and the very best restaurants were wheelchair accessible. At the zoo, the wheelchair let us bypass the long queues to the most popular animals, and we pretended that Dave needed one more than the allotted attendant (his cap turned over his ear, which made him look feebleminded), moving so fast that we raced right past the pandas, until we realized, oh, and then we backed up respectfully and looked at them looking at us. We laughed constantly.

Back in Los Angeles, we went to the gospel brunch at the House of Blues and had such an easy, good time that we came back the next night to hear Tom Jones, which was not so easy. The so-called wheelchair area was behind a wall of standing people, and when I confronted one tall blonde, who stood herself right in front of Dave, she wailed, but I can't see, and I snapped back, well he can't walk. There are photos of that Christmas—Quinn as Santa Claus on Dave's lap, our goofy Hawaiian New Year's Eve party, with the whole family in loud shirts drinking fruity cocktails. Sara and I performed "Climb Every Mountain" even though no one had requested it.

By the end of the ten days, I was exhausted. I started crying as I packed up Dave's things and I cried all the way to the airport in something like a mini-nervous breakdown. But we remembered this trip as a good one.

For the next six months Dave went nowhere, except up and down the promenade with Dobie, occasionally to

141

my house for Sunday brunch or dinner. In the spring, Sara and I took him for a day at Niagara Falls, where we had been together as children. It was a celebration of his fiftieth birthday. We had a picnic in the park and then donned plastic capes and took the elevator down under the cliff, to a cavelike opening directly across from the falls, where we could see the *Maid of the Mist* making its stately turns directly below us, and we shouted and laughed into the vapor and thunder of the falls.

TRAVELING TO Los Angeles gave Dave the courage to plan a cruise. Online, I found him a travel agent in California, who specialized in helping disabled travelers; Debbie was herself disabled and she got Dave to undertake a twelve-week, around-the-world millennium cruise on the Holland America ship MS *Rotterdam*. (Debbie and I spoke on the phone a number of times, and she also talked to Dave; she had exactly the right personality to persuade him to commit to this daunting trip, as it was very costly, and Dave, like Dad, was congenitally frugal.) Over the spring and summer of 1999, he began to prepare, slowly and deliberately, for this adventure, which would embark from Florida in January 2000.

But also over this period, he slid into a cycle of not drinking enough fluids and becoming constipated and weak. It was a truth we silently acknowledged but could not explore that Dave's condition would usually deteriorate on the eve of my leaving Toronto for any length of time and that he would suffer a health crisis while I was away. I could not persuade him to see a doctor regularly or to institute a permanent home care arrangement. He would not pay for medical assistance. The rules governing home care in Ontario at that time were incomprehensible, and there were mysterious bureaucratic glitches, which we always failed to anticipate, that would mean that no nurse would come to visit or that he would have to apply over and over again, and sometimes a nurse would come from one agency and sometimes from another. The Participation service in his building did not provide nursing care, only something euphemistically termed "assisted living," and this service too was erratic and unpredictable; the staff were terribly underpaid and poorly trained, and good people did not stay long. (One night early in Dave's stay at Windward, two young men scarcely past adolescence arrived at his door, eager to help, armed with rubber tubing and a booklet about how to catheterize.) When his spiral into illness began, with prolonged constipation and bladder problems, the Participation staff urged him to just take "lots" of a powerful laxative.

His voice was softer and weaker, and he had numerous moments of hopelessness: he could not get into bed on his own, and he was frequently catheterizing himself but he would run out of lubricant. He would have no quarters for his laundry. He decided to cut back on baclofen, the drug he took for spasticity, because it was expensive, so he became very stiff. He could not stand by the toilet, and when I returned after a month away doing research for a book, we

143

did not discuss how long it had been since he had urinated standing up. He was catheterizing himself more often than he would admit. This meant: sterilizing a catheter in a small Pyrex jug of water, in the microwave in the kitchen. Carrying the catheter in the jug of boiled water on his lap in his wheelchair into the bathroom. Disinfecting his right hand and penis with soap and water, using only that hand, as his left arm and hand were by then useless. With his right hand, putting lubricant onto the catheter, inserting the catheter...

He had no friends of his own, in Toronto, and in any case he would never ask anyone for help. He resisted using the services that Participation could provide and when he was in dire need always tried to solve the problem himself before he called anyone. He was an unreliable witness to his own condition, especially when it was exacerbated by circumstances he chose to ignore, like flu symptoms or stiffness and pain. He had a desultory relationship with a GP he seldom saw. He drove himself into corners of panic and helplessness, because he was too stubborn to ask for help.

The three of us planned a two-week holiday at a cottage in August, and Lorne was to join us as well. There are very few wheelchair-accessible cottages in Ontario, I learned, over several weeks of doing research, phoning, and driving to look at places. But I advertised in newspapers and found a large house on Pigeon Lake near Peterborough, where, as part of an exorbitant rent, the owner agreed to install a temporary ramp through the garage into the house, for access to the living and dining and kitchen areas on the upper level, and there were bedrooms and a bathroom on the lower level, accessible from a deck.

The day we were to head north, Dave was weak, could barely speak, and had a high temperature and sharp pains in his arms. He later admitted to double vision and some confusion. He went by ambulance to St. Mike's and was in the emergency room for almost seven hours. Sara and I ignored the suggestion of the admitting clerk and sat with him in his stall. It was like a garage, a series of bays separated by skimpy curtains: the woman in the next bay was choking on her vomit; the man two curtains down had a ruptured stomach and was spurting blood all over the floor; and somewhere nearby someone died while Dave was waiting to be seen. Dave perked up very suddenly after a dose of antibiotic, and we went home.

We delayed our departure for two days. The next morning he was feeling terrible, with more chills, thick, dark urine, and a panicky look in his eyes. The van and driver had been rebooked. Rita, the new St. Elizabeth's nurse, took charge, as Sara and I were unsure what to do. Rita called Dave's doctor and asked her to check the lab results right away and change the antibiotic. We decided that catheterizing was the main issue and discussed my doing this, with Dave, which he grudgingly accepted. (His method had become very suspect—he used paper towels and a bar of soap slipping through one hand—and he may have infected himself this way.) Also from Rita, a long, stern lecture about fluids, the one I had been giving him for months. But he would not hear, or rather accept,

145

the truth of this advice, stuck in a rationale about how drinking made him pee and he was unable to get up at night. To Rita he admitted that he had been taking Metamucil, but with not enough water. He had much invested in being "fine" until suddenly he was not. I told him that it was either drink or die, that he would end up in hospital dehydrated. Bruce, the very best attendant from Participation, who adored Dave's dog, Dobie, told me that he had put Dave to bed on Saturday after his return from hospital and that he was virtually crying from pain. We never saw him cry.

Miraculously, by noon on Tuesday, we were on the road, Dave driven in the van with enormous quantities of essentials, including his electric wheelchair and big electrified recliner, the bedside pole, a toilet seat, an extra manual wheelchair, medical supplies, and Dobie; Sara and I driving in my car with a new prescription, the ramps, the food and wine, and three computers. Lorne met us at the house we had rented.

Dave was a nervous wreck at first. Shouting, groaning, keening over the slightest thing; Lorne got up three times with him in the first night. We were sterilizing catheters in the middle of night and discreetly lubricating and setting up more sterile conditions for him. We made him drink gallons, more than he realized—cranberry juice, ginger ale, water. The rhythm took time to establish: drink, drink, floods of urine, change of clothing, towels, laundry, laundry, laundry, all the bedding changed every morning, the recliner and wheelchair sponged down with antiseptic spray, a new kind of Depends with straps that he refused to use at first, whining and keening and hollering, and then lectures about shouting, because on the first night Sara found him near collapse, shouting for help, but we thought he was just shouting in frustration as he often did. Lectures also about deep breathing, when he would get into a painful need to pee but could not.

Over the eleven long days and nights, he stopped using the catheter (about the fourth day), his appetite leapt up enormously, and he ate heartily. He went from not being able to pee at night without a catheter to not being able to pee at night unless he stood to release it to peeing copiously lying down, through the night, but without pain. It was not possible to figure out how much of this peeing was voluntary or otherwise. It seemed we talked of nothing else, smelled nothing else, saw nothing but soaked shorts and underwear on the bathroom floor and a great heavy diaper in the wastebasket. We took turns sleeping downstairs, close to him, and even so we all woke up every morning exhausted, feeling like we were starting duty. We cooked, did laundry, poured drinks, looked after Dobie, monitored the drugs, which he easily forgot.

147

But the semblance of normalcy slowly returned. He took Dobie for long stately walks, leash attached to wheelchair, through the woods and down the gravel road to Elim Lodge for the newspaper every morning. I persuaded him to increase the baclofen dose from one a day to three, and his muscles relaxed. A softness returned to his body; he could mostly get up, only needed help swinging his feet up into bed. His keening subsided, and there was hardly any shouting. His voice got stronger. He worked on the software on the laptop he had bought for his cruise.

I never lost my temper or raised my voice. I had to walk away from the roaring, which pounded through me like nails. But as I ran up and down stairs, shopped endlessly for medical, dog, food stuff, washed the dog for fleas, washed the dog again, moved lamps, brought drinks, prepared three tempting meals a day, did more laundry, helped him on with his shorts, pulling up the Depends surreptitiously, I could imagine, with shame and fear, how abuse could happen in such situations. If you were trapped for months and years in caregiving, with no relief, no help, with a patient who was far more challenged than Dave mentally and physically, it would be hard to remain serene, and oh, God, that is a profound understatement. And he wanted so fiercely not to be dependent, to do everything himself, not to share every detail of his peeing and shitting and sleeping or not and feeling better or worse, tired or strong, on and on and on it went. By the time we left for home I, selfishly, wanted my life back.

I can still hear the clicking, all night long, of Ping-Pong balls, because at first Lorne and Sara played maniacally, when we would all be up most of the night. After the first few days they did not play anymore, and we learned to ration our attentiveness, one person at a time. We were a round-the-clock nursing service, and it was not clear to what extent Dave knew this; or was it necessary for his dignity and even survival that he not acknowledge what we were doing? He did not say much; we could see him trying to be patient, trying not to roar, trying to be good-natured and pleasant in the night. How he must have hated to lie there, shouting Marian or Sara or Lorne.

When we did small, joyous things, like taking a bottle of champagne down to the lake for Sara's belated birthday celebration or throwing a stick into the lake for Dobie to retrieve or having a bonfire and roasting marshmallows in the fire pit, we snapped back into our comfortable sibling triangle. Sara told the terrible jokes of her Georgian aesthetician in Toronto, and we shared a Botsford perspective on our decidedly odd host (who hovered nearby in a trailer) and this huge, strange, sterile house that we were in, and we laughed and took photos and talked about our childhood and the summerhouse and where Dave would be going on the *Rotterdam*.

I looked at the calm spread of lake, the family of loons that hovered always at the end of dock, even when I was swimming, the deep shadow of mature trees on the lawn in mid-afternoon, at the moon shimmering on water in deep of night when I was up helping him.

And how will he manage on his three-month, around-the-world millennium cruise was the question that simmered beneath the surface.

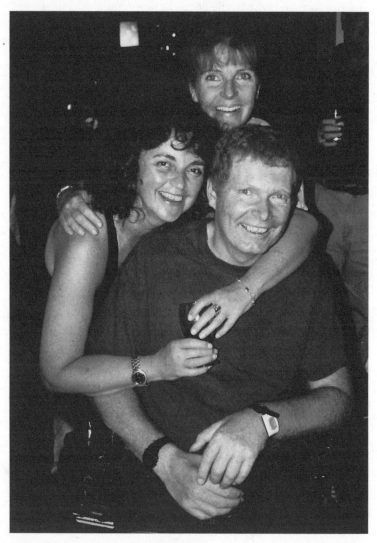

Sara, Dave, and I at the summerhouse

4

DAVE

AT

SEA

AFTER lunch, there is a pause, as we had agreed that we would "do the ashes" at three o'clock. The wind blows in hot gusts at times, and the skein of cloud slides on and off the sun. Jonathan and Sara go down to the beach to fish; Jon catches a tiny pike and throws it back. Katherine and Gideon doze. Suki goes to the point with Quinn and they swim and Quinn worries about leeches. I sit with Lorne under one of the big spruce trees. He has confessed that he was nervous about this day, not sure what to expect. But we're doing all of this with Dave, and that means companionable silence, a few good decisions, some jokes, a beer or two, and more silence.

I bring out the cedar boxes from the tapestry bag and set them out under the trees. After Dave's death he was cremated in a plain pine box (unexpectedly, I'd had to choose between solid wood and particleboard, just for burning), and then his ashes remained for a couple of weeks at the funeral home in Toronto. I was bothered by how we would transport the ashes for this ceremony of scattering on Lake Beaverhouse, and then by what would happen to such a receptacle after we had scattered the ashes. I didn't know what people did. When our parents died ten years earlier, their ashes had come to us in thick plastic bags in plain black and white cardboard boxes. I had decided that Dave's ashes needed a wooden container. But the container would only be for holding the ashes until they were scattered, and if there was only one, who would keep it? So there had to be two wooden boxes, one for Sara and one for me. I looked in craft shops and antique shops and art stores in Toronto, not sure what I was looking for, except that the boxes had to honor Dave's love and skill of woodworking.

Two weeks after Dave's death, Sara and I went for the weekend to Niagara-on-the-Lake, where Rita Brown, the mother of Sara's partner, Chris Brown, lived. I explained my quixotic quest to Rita. "Why don't we have a quick look in the little antique shops in St. David's, just down the road?" she suggested.

The first thing I saw when I walked into the first shop was a small oblong cedar box, sitting on the corner of a display table inside the door. It was a miniature hope chest, a salesman's sample made to be taken door to door, most probably between the wars in communities across Ontario. It was nine inches long, four inches tall, with solid brass hinges and catch, and with some carved detail and a well-burnished finish. On the inside of the cover there was a stamp saying Lane Cedar Chests, and on the bottom, an old paper label naming "... echtels Limited—Hanover, Ontario" as the Canadian maker of "the Famous Lane Cedar Chests... since 1864." The price was $45.

As I breathed in the sweet cedar aroma that still emanated from the little chest, I glanced at the other end of the display table, and there sat an identical box.

In my basement in Toronto, I had the two handsome teak tool boxes the size of real hope chests that Dave had made fifteen years earlier and brought with him when he moved from Campbell River out east to the summerhouse. These little cedar boxes somehow acknowledged those chests. I went to the funeral home, where Dave's ashes were measured into two small bags and placed into the cedar boxes.

Lorne, who shared Dave's passion for woodworking, now looks at the boxes closely, reads the label. "Oh," he says suddenly. "I know this name. I taught the son of this cabinetmaker; he was from St. Catharine's." For some reason, this recognition relaxes Lorne.

Sara comes over with a beer, and she and I show Lorne the photos in the album; there is one of Dave and Lorne and their heavily loaded canoe, on this camping spot, in 1994, and many others of him in boats. And skiing, cycling, scuba diving with Kathy, fishing and hiking and camping, often with Lorne.

To a great degree, Dave's life was defined by his body, by physical skill and dexterity. He had a particular kind of long-legged grace, especially when he was in motion. He was a tall, good-looking, broad-shouldered man and must have drawn glances on the ski hills; he went often to Whistler and Blackcomb and sometimes to Colorado to ski.

"He was such a good skier, eh?" Lorne says.

"When did he stop? I last saw him ski in . . . was it 1990?"

"Yeah, me too," says Sara, laughing. "When we all had New Year's together at Big White. Remember how he got really mad at us when we tried to pick out women for him to dance with?"

"But he must've skied after that . . . "

"I know exactly when it was," says Sara. "After our first summer at the summerhouse. So . . . 1993? He went back to Campbell River and went to Whistler as usual that winter. But when he rode right up to the top of the mountain, for his last run of the day, he realized he did not have the strength to ski down."

"So he took the chairlift down again . . . "

"He must have hated that," says Lorne. He closes the album.

DAVE'S PREPARATIONS for his millennium cruise became a joint project in the fall of 1999, and we planned that I would go with him for the first five days, to get him set up on the ship. When I arrived at Dave's apartment the night before his departure, he was in high anxiety mode. He dropped a Pyrex cup on the bathroom floor shortly after I arrived—glass everywhere. The nurse had not been to change the burn dressing on his leg (from boiling water when he was sterilizing a catheter), and he was exhausted, with deep pains in his shoulders and upper arms. He could not transfer alone, from wheelchair to recliner or toilet or bed. He panicked in the bathroom when I tried to help; I started calling Home Care for a nurse. Dobie was running around in circles, knowing something was about to happen.

I packed and labeled everything with Holland America Line (HAL) baggage tags; Dave would be on the ship for twelve weeks. The itinerary included the Caribbean, Antarctica, the coast of Africa, Japan, China, and Hawaii and all the oceans in between. He needed winter and summer clothing, including a linen sport coat and several ties. I had had buttons taken off all his shirts and pants and replaced with Velcro. He had a small microwave oven for sterilizing catheters, a bulky toilet seat wrapped in black garbage bags, a car battery charger for the wheelchair, medication for three months, and hundreds of catheters and dozens of tubes of KY jelly and boxes of gauze pads. A letter from his doctor to the ship's doctor, prescriptions and a health care power of attorney, a huge world atlas, a bird book, a laptop computer loaded with voice-recognition software, binoculars, digital camera, portable disc player and CDs, power bar, extension cords, phone cord, a tool kit with screwdrivers and batteries and electrical and duct tape. He had purchased a second-hand hospital bed and electric recliner chair by phone from a store in Fort Lauderdale, and these would be delivered to the ship and installed in his cabin.

Two nurses finally showed up. Rita was Dave's favorite; Christine had never been there before. The three of us loomed over Dave in the small bathroom. Rita took his temperature and changed his bandage. Christine stood with arms folded and asked: Why are you in a wheelchair? Why didn't they give you a hit of steroids for your trip? Have you been to the MS assessment center? Do you do exercises? She was Germanic, tough, aggressive. Rita was Jamaican, warm, and she could make Dave laugh. She told us an elaborate story about a home care nurse who also worked most winters as a cruise prostitute. She looked at the doctor's letter, snorted as she showed it to Christine, and added more details about Dave's symptoms and recurring concerns; they agreed that he did not have a good, activist doctor. Dave endured this intense attention without comment.

As we stood chatting in the bathroom, Bruce from Participation came to take Dobie, to stay with him while Dave was away. "Sit, please," said Bruce firmly. Dave did not say goodbye or pet Dobie or make any sign whatsoever of affection. He wheeled himself silently into his bedroom, afraid of crying.

Before I left that evening, Dave made several changes to his will and signed the health care power of attorney, which I had insisted that he make and that he take with him on the cruise. It stated that either Sara or I had be consulted in the case of any medical intervention anywhere in the world. In spite of his agitation, he had read both documents thoroughly. His changes to the will were small, syntactical, to make sure that Sara and I were treated equally. Close to midnight, two Participation workers came to the apartment to witness his signatures.

When I came back at 4:45 the next morning, with a van and a calm young driver, Dave was again swearing in the bathroom and eating handfuls of dry cereal. His voice was high, strained, but we amicably managed the next five hours of driving, baggage-handling, airports, customs, and the plane trip. In Miami we were met by Holland America, and Dave's luggage and paraphernalia were whisked away, but there was a 45-minute wait for his wheelchair, which arrived with a broken joystick. We took a bus to the Fort Lauderdale docks and were directed to the head of the line of nine hundred passengers waiting to get on the ship. As we boarded we were caught by the ship's photographer; Dave looks stiff and rather grim, with a perky Dutch maiden—emblematic of the Holland in Holland America—nestling in beside his knees. I am wild eyed and grinning maniacally. We made our way into the bowels of the ship and were in Cabin 1804 on Dolphin Deck One by 1:00 p.m.

The first thing I saw was that the hospital bed and electric recliner chair he had purchased for the trip had arrived and been assembled, in the middle of the cabin. Next: there were no windows, only two tiny, distant portholes at the end of a narrow recessed box. The room was small and dark. There was an empty alcove where the bed might fit, but it would require a carpenter to squeeze it in. The luggage arrived, and we piled everything in the middle of the room; it was not clear where I would be sleeping, although Dave had paid for my five nights on the ship.

This cabin was billed as "wheelchair accessible," which we quickly realized did not mean *electric*-wheelchair accessible. All the doors were heavy, and they did not stay open; it was impossible for Dave to open a door from his chair. His

North American toilet seat did not fit the European toilet. The bathroom was very small, with no room to turn. I could hear him swearing and moaning from the corridor, where I waited, as he would not let me help him. I heard one, two, three catheters being opened, covered with lubricant, discarded. He fell, crashing to the floor; I ran back into the room and pulled the emergency cord. The phone instantly rang and I answered, to be told that only if it rang five times without being answered would the stewards know there was a real emergency and respond. Two stewards arrived and slowly picked Dave up; it was clear this task was not one of their accustomed chores.

Once this crisis passed, we had lunch in a cafeteria, undertook with some confusion and amusement the compulsory fire and lifeboat drill with life jackets, went to the cast-off reception, and spent a couple of hours exploring the ship.

The *Rotterdam* was an enormous and glamorous ship, beautifully finished, with sweeping public spaces and also myriad rooms and spaces for solitude or privacy, something nine hundred people might crave occasionally over a twelve-week journey. The lowest level, A deck, was the crew deck and tender service, where guests rarely went. Dolphin Deck One consisted of cabins and the infirmary, which was just down the corridor from Dave's cabin. Deck Two had more cabins, and Deck Three had a broad, sheltered wooden promenade that went all the way around the boat, a place for Dave to motor along and get shaded fresh air, but without automated doors, so he would have to wait until someone was there to help him enter and exit. Deck Four held the front office, shops (selling everything from toothpaste to sequined evening gowns), the small, pretty Odyssey dining room and the Queen's Show Lounge, with deep, soft chairs and a stage for academic lecturers by day and can-can girls by night. Deck Five, the upper promenade, featured the grand La Fontaine dining room and lots of little bars and dance floors, and a library, the Explorer lounge, Internet café, and a huge electronic map, where the *Rotterdam*'s route was charted with blinking lights. Deck Six was the Verandah, where most cabins had a tiny private balcony. Deck Seven was navigation, the bridge, some penthouse suites, and an open saltwater pool at the stern, my favorite place on the ship. Deck Eight held the Lido restaurant, bars, spa, a very large pool with whirlpools, and outdoor bars. Deck Nine was the sports deck, with shuffleboard, and the Crow's Nest bar, also an excellent observation spot.

When Dave was ready to get into bed, we called the front desk for assistance; 45 minutes later, a steward arrived reluctantly with a clean sheet, having been told Dave had had an accident. He was helped into bed after midnight. He had been up for more than 20 hours.

The room was in chaos, nothing unpacked because his bed blocked one closet and the second was behind the bathroom door, which we had propped open. The air conditioning was not working, and we got a small, noisy fan. I found a spare mattress in the corridor and dragged it in to sleep on the floor. We were both exhausted, and we did not talk about the daunting prospect of twelve weeks for him in this space. I would be on the ship for four more days.

THERE WAS a deep, dark stain of blood on Dave's sheet
when he got out of bed the next morning. He had a huge,
black, bursting mole high on his back. We had breakfast
in the main dining room, and while Dave went to the doctor, I took a list of issues to the front desk and waited in a
long line; there were many people with picayune problems,
not unexpected, with nine hundred retired, affluent, and
seasoned travelers. I finally spoke to Suzanne, the guest
relations manager. I was polite as I went through my list of
problems with cabin 1804. It had not occurred to me to ask
for a cabin change, but the possibility of this option emerged
during the conversation. Suzanne said she would call head
office in Seattle, but because it was Friday she was not sure
she would be able to connect. I sent a fax to Debbie, Dave's
travel agent in Los Angeles.

When I got back to the cabin, Dave had returned from
the infirmary. The mole? I asked. The doctor said it should
be excised but that it was not an emergency. As the nurses
dressed it, they talked casually of taking him off the ship
at Buenos Aires, the first port where he might see a doctor,
in four weeks' time. At what enormous cost, we wondered.
This ship was American; it cost $50 for one brief consulta-
tion and dressing.

Dave was sitting in the recliner, facing the tiny portholes,
like two paper towel rolls at the end of a tunnel. He stood,
slowly, to transfer to his wheelchair. He said very quietly, "I
think I've been sold a bill of goods." There were tears in his
eyes.

Let's go up to the pool, I said.

I swam, and we had lunch; it was wonderfully hot and sunny and the sea was blue, the breeze salt-scented. I came back to the cabin alone to call Debbie and Sara, barely able to speak. Suzanne came with a carpenter, who said yes, the bed would fit in the alcove. The room looked like a hurricane zone, with stuff piled everywhere. I, the rottweiler, could not stop crying as we spoke. Suzanne said, let's wait to hear from Seattle.

Dave and I went to a lecture on the history of the Caribbean in the theater, and he relaxed suddenly, intent on gathering knowledge. When we returned to the cabin, Sara phoned from Los Angeles; she had spoken with Holland America, threatened lawyers and press coverage, and told them we would "pull Dave off the ship," with *huge* publicity. Dave and I had several moments of hysterical laughter, imagining a press conference on the ship, with CNN helicopters, hovering...We could only wait, so we got fully, formally dressed and went to the captain's champagne reception and dinner. In the La Fontaine dining room Dave was assigned to a table with six other people, two gentle Midwestern couples and two older, quite shy single women. The food was what one would expect at any high-end hotel. The charming waiter made it seem that removing foot rests from a wheelchair and cutting meat were things he was born to do. We made pleasant conversation and relaxed.

Most people on the ship were much older than Dave and much richer; after dinner, we caught a glimpse inside several penthouse suites on Deck Seven—vast rooms cluttered with leather trunks, champagne buckets, and big baskets of roses. There were some notable eccentrics on board: a skinny old man named Baba Loo, who hovered and floated around the front desk and talked to everyone he made eye contact with; a tiny woman who wore enormous felt flowerpot and watermelon hats, a different one each day (she might also have been quite blind). There were a number of people in manual wheelchairs (with patient spouses to push them everywhere) and two or three with small, streamlined scooters, but Dave was the only passenger in an electric wheelchair. One frail-looking woman walked briskly, hauling her oxygen tank on wheels behind her. There were diabetics and people who shook all the time, people who were deaf, and some who were perhaps not quite sound mentally.

There were also heavy smokers and hard drinkers, compulsive gamblers, and people with black tans and gold jewelry and hard-edged minds. I overheard a conversation poolside between two men who were finding China a damn fine place to do business, because they could move people wherever and whenever they felt like it and no irritating environmental permits were ever required.

In the theater that evening we listened to Pat Boone sing in his white sport coat, and then we wandered around the ship. This long after-dinner time seemed pointless to me, because people were drinking and dancing and shopping and gambling and we were not. We were in a floating social bubble, a tightly ranked hierarchy of white, privileged people graciously tended to by Filipino and Indonesian staff.

The ship's officers were white and Dutch, the other senior personnel mostly white and American. We stood in front of the map with the blinking lights as the ship moved silently, effortlessly, south into the smooth Caribbean Sea.

From my mattress on the floor that night, I listened to Dave as he slept and resisted the urge to offer to help him when he got up in the night. He was recalibrating his methods of daily living. He had no floor-to-ceiling pole to help him pivot getting in and out of bed. The control pad for the bed had to be placed where he could always touch it. He had to determine exactly where on the bed rail to place his right hand and how, if at all, his stiff left arm could be used as a support. The wheelchair footrests had to be lifted out of the way before he could get into or out of the chair. His wheelchair had to be set at night at precisely the correct angle beside the bed so that he could swivel into it once he was standing. He had to be able to reach the joystick to bring the chair an inch or two closer, then change the angle ever so slightly so that there was a place for his left hand to land. If ever he lost his balance and crashed like a felled tree to the floor, the emergency cord had to be within his reach. He did the same calculations with his reclining chair and with the toilet seat in the bathroom. We had come to take for granted the many small things that supported him at home—a MedAlert bracelet, two speaker phones, a bath chair, precisely placed handrails, remote controls for doors. This little cabin in the depths of a ship crossing oceans was an unforgiving space for a silent and stubborn man, alone for twelve weeks.

People wondered: why didn't I go with him for the whole trip? Spending money and admitting that he needed help were not things Dave did easily. The trip was the most expensive thing he had ever undertaken, and to take me or someone else would have cost the same again. Also, he was determined to make this journey on his own.

The next morning I was up before eight o'clock and out looking for Suzanne. She took me to look at two possible cabins, one on the main deck with a narrow, boxed-in entry, and then 6104 on the Verandah deck. She opened the door, and I was struck with how much light filled the room. It was a suite-sized cabin, an open rectangle design, with a large bay window, which had a light metal staircase outside in front of it, the reason this was not an actual "verandah" suite and presumably why it had not been sold. Dave saw the room after breakfast with a carpenter, who made notes of his needs, including the removal of the bathroom door. Both the bed and chair could be set up to see out the window, the closets were easily reached, and there was lots of turning room and a sofa bed for my remaining two nights. Suddenly everyone and everything was focused on this problem; the head of housekeeping was there to oversee the move, and Dave was in his new cabin before noon.

In the blistering midafternoon heat, I went ashore at Grand Cayman Island, where in the little port town you can buy diamonds, emeralds, Rolex watches, but there is no grocery store. I found a dusty variety store and bought a plastic laundry basket, some Advil, a thermometer, two plastic microwave containers for sterilizing the catheters. I

stumbled around the hot, ugly town, in and out of shops. I
came upon a deserted courtyard, with a large noisy fountain in full tumult in the center of the small square. I sat on
a wooden bench close to the fountain and cried, huge, rack-
ing sobs, for several minutes.

I returned to the ship and set up the room: power bar,
extension cords (for bed and chair), phone extension cord—
duct tape, electrician's tape, screwdrivers all in play. I organized the closets and put catheters and gauze pads in the
bathroom and set up the microwave and battery charger
and computer, rigged a belt around the handle of the state-
room door so that Dave could easily get out, and unlocked
the door permanently so that he could always get back in.
Security was a luxury he could not afford. I tried to engage
with Dave's steward, a shy, serious Filipino named Eko, who
appeared to absorb the information I saturated him with
but who never smiled; he seemed either afraid of or nervous
about Dave. There was no connection, no visible compassion or humor.

We had dinner in the small Odyssey dining room on the
fourth deck. A harmonica player doodled in the corner, and
we had excellent wine and relaxed conversation about our
past travels. We lifted a glass to the Rocky Defile on the
Coppermine River.

Later I danced one dance with one of the eight "gentlemen hosts," dapper, white-haired men in blue blazers and
white trousers whose sole job was to ask single women to
dance in the evenings. My gentleman host was slim and
balding, and he steered me with a firm, light hand on the

small of my back. He was from North Carolina, he said, a widower, and this transoceanic outing was his fourth as a dancing partner. He was obliged to spread his services around, and he could only dance one dance at a time with each woman. Relationships were not approved, he assured me solemnly as he bowed slightly and thanked me for the dance. I wondered why there were eight gentlemen hosts who did nothing but dance and only three stewards on duty at night for the whole ship. And why there was no specialist in services for the disabled. And why a passenger could pay someone extra to do their hair or laundry but not to provide extra assistance with dressing or getting in and out of bed.

That night, Dave got into bed himself. He had worked out the essential calibrations; for every task there was an engineer's solution. My pullout sofa bed seemed luxurious after two nights on the floor, and through the window I could see the night sky.

WE BOTH experienced these days on a ship as one long blur, brought into minimal focus by the daily schedule delivered nightly to the cabin, often with little extras like robes, pens, a traveling clock, glossy books. It was like going to camp, and there were people on the ship who had traveled together before, greeting one another with hysterical excitement like return campers and displaying some air of smug familiarity with the ship and its routines. Other people were confused, like us, standing in front of elevators, not sure where they were, exactly, or if they wanted to go up or down. People had glazed looks and on Sunday morning a bit of a stagger; it was moderately rough. I got seasickness tabs for Dave from the dispensary. He set up his computer voicing attachments and visited the Internet café. From his first days of planning his trip, he had a fierce determination to write and send a regular cruise log to family and friends, and he was trying to figure out how to do this.

I ascended to the saltwater pool on the stern lip of Deck Seven, had a leisurely swim, and talked with a woman my age from Toronto, who also saw everyone as very old and spoiled and very rich. I was actively seeking people who might befriend Dave after I departed. In the afternoon he and I went to a lecture and "flagship forum" on the upcoming handover of the Panama Canal. (There had been a vets' meeting in the morning, and clearly there were many ex-navy/military types on board.) The moderator managed to find an even split in the vote on the potentially heated topic, a canny piece of diplomacy; these people were to be bound together for three months.

The trip through the Panama Canal, a momentous journey through landscape and history, would take the *Rotterdam* almost twelve hours, from the Atlantic to Panama City on the Pacific side. The entire day would be a privileged window on exceptional feats of engineering, and Dave, his head brimming with information and questions, was on deck by seven, carefully lifted out by one of the food stewards, who already knew his name. It was already hot; the light shimmered, the air was heavy on the skin. There were stations set up with coffee and sweet rolls and an expert positioned on the bridge with the captain to give a commentary most of the day.

There was a serious sense of occasion as we approached the first set of locks. The MS *Rotterdam* is almost 800 feet long and 106 feet wide; among the passengers there was anxiety about whether or not the ship would be able to scrape through and a feeling of somehow being part of the effort to do so. Small engines on railway tracks, called donkeys, were clipped by hand onto the ship with long, thick cables, and they slowly, smoothly pulled the ship the length of the lock. From the deck it looked as if there was less than a foot's clearance on either side. We murmured appreciatively as the ship glided through.

By noon the deck burned underfoot and the railing was too hot to touch. People drifted in and out; Dave spent the afternoon in the Crow's Nest, where it was cool and quiet and where he could see the canal and hear the commentary. He said very little, absorbing every detail. I could see that he was profoundly pleased by this day.

I packed my bag and wrote notes to chief steward Bambang and to the people next door (about Dave's keening, as they shared his bathroom wall) and notes to Dave, reminding him not to keen and holler if he could help it. I poked steam holes in the microwave containers; told Eko more, more, more; left a generous tip for him; talked to Bambang to get him to talk to Eko. Then I got down on my knees beside the sofa bed and prayed.

I prayed that Dave would be able to manage all those tiny calibrations that he relied on.

I prayed that he would never fall down in the middle of the night out of reach of the telephone.

168

I prayed that people would befriend him and that he wouldn't lose his temper with staff and that the people next door were kind people.

I prayed like someone who did not really know how to pray.

Shortly after five, Dave and I descended to A Deck for my departure. We walked past the huge barracks and dining area for crew, a world scarcely imagined or glimpsed by passengers immersed in their pleasures and discontents. I hugged Dave twice, and tried, without success, not to cry. Thanks, he muttered. He was rigid as stone.

"So Dave," I said (in our dry family way), "on a scale of one to ten, how confident are you about this trip?"

"Five," he replied instantly with the glimmer of a smile.

I climbed down a wobbly rope ladder onto a small boat and roared away to shore, spent the night in a frigid, musty room in a cheap Panama City motel and was back in Toronto the next afternoon.

. . .

Tuesday, January 11, 2000
From: mbf@istar.ca
To: dbotsford@interhop.net

Dave, it takes about two hours to fly from Panama City to Miami. It's just after six, and I'm already home. Hope you're fine; it was a tough four days, but you're set up as best as possible, and now you just need some luck. If you can't find stuff, or are confused about anything, let me know. If your cabin service isn't good, speak to Bambang.

Oh, a lovely, bosomy blonde Dutch woman named Ramona was on the shuttle boat at Panama; she is off the ship for five days in Galápagos, gets back on at one of the Peru stops. She wrote down your name and cabin number and said she'd be talking to you. She is gorgeous, friendly . . .

Tell nurse Lorraine that I mailed her letters in Miami. She is from Alaska.

Lots of love, Mare.

. . .

IT WAS a cold winter in Toronto. I would go down to Dave's apartment regularly, water his plants, sit at his desk staring out at frozen Lake Ontario and visualize him on the ship. The apartment was silent and sterile without Dobie and all of Dave's paraphernalia. I got the place cleaned and brought in a contractor to fix the walls bashed by the wheelchair. I had the *Rotterdam* daily schedule open beside the computer, so I knew every day what he might or might not do: Caribbean theme dinner, probably. Black and White Officers' Ball, unlikely, and where would they have a ball? I sent e-mails almost every day, which he often did not respond to, because his system was incompatible with the ship's, because the Internet café manager had to retype his notes, because it cost $15 to check his e-mail. I called the ship but often did not get through; I finally figured out that the satellite was down whenever the ship was in port. I told Dave he'd be pleased to know it would cost even more for me to phone the ship from shore ($16 per minute) than it would the other way. I sent faxes, hoping they would end up under his door.

A week, two weeks passed. Cryptic e-mails from Dave on the Chilean coast: "Hi, Mare... I've managed to get off the ship a couple times. I usually need help on the steep gangway ramps but it's not bad. In Valparaiso, Chile today. It's definitely getting cooler as we go south. I plan to get off and look around after I charge my chair. Stretch my legs, heh, heh... The nurse has been changing my bandage every couple days and not charging me..."

I followed Dave's progress on a map of South America. I sent him hearty, hectoring notes: "Sounds like you're having fun. Enjoy that 25 percent upgrade!!!"

"Tomorrow night: Dutch Theme Dinner."

"Do you have what you need for the doctor in Buenos Aires? You know where your wallet/health card and keys are? Make sure someone will stay with you THE WHOLE TIME..."

"Your cruise log is great!"

"Oh, it's really, really cold here, 20 and 30 below, and nasty winds and everyone is sick. So keep going!"

FROM DAVE'S cruise log, sent to family and friends:

. . .

Punta Arenas, Chile; January 25, 2000: I am using my voice recognition software and laptop computer to write this. The software is handy but I tend to make a lot of errors, so you will have to excuse all of the weird mistakes. Since I seldom use it I am not very good at corrections.

I started in Fort Lauderdale Jan. 6 with sister Marian accompanying me as far as the Pacific side of the Panama

Canal. The ship then sailed down the west coast of South America with stops at various cities in Peru, Ecuador, and Chile. We are now about to sail across the Drake Channel and visit the northern peninsula of Antarctica. There is a bevy of prominent lecturers on-board, so I am getting my fill of information about Antarctica and South America.

This city called Punta Arenas (pop. 110,000) is on the Strait of Magellan about halfway through. The strait is much wider than I expected it to be. I thought a ship the size of the *Rotterdam* would be bouncing off the walls of the channel, but in fact in this area there are great distances between its shores (several kilometers). We are now sailing to another city, Ushuaia, "the southernmost city in the world" and will arrive tomorrow morning. The next few days should be very interesting as we sail to Antarctica and go through several spectacular channels along the west coast of the Antarctica peninsula. There is also an iceberg the size of Rhode Island that we should see on our way back.

I had some difficulty setting up the e-mailing process. I cannot use my cabin telephone because the satellite and my computer modems will not talk to each other properly, so this letter is somewhat later than I planned. I have to save it on a floppy disk and take it to our ship's Internet manager. I plan to send an update every few weeks.

Ushuaia, Argentina; January 26: On the south shore of Tierra Del Fuego. Cool clear weather here today. I left the ship for about an hour and traveled around the wharf and the streets for a short while. The streets are not generally wheelchair accessible; no way of getting on and off the sidewalk at the street crossings, so it is rather difficult to travel.

Cape Horn, Chile; January 27: We stopped in front of Cape Horn for about an hour early this morning. It is very soupy today. The weather here can become extremely stormy at any time. We are now headed south to Antarctica across the Drake channel. It is still very foggy but not too rough . . . yet.

   We just completed a lifeboat drill, mandatory on cruise ships at least once per week. I showed up in bare feet and got a lot of strange looks, but I am used to traveling around in bare feet in this type of weather, so who cares.

Antarctica; January 28 and 29: Awoke this morning to calm seas, and clear skies, rock, ice, and snow everywhere it seems. We had sailed across Drake Passage during the night. It's a different world here after all the dreary fog around Cape Horn. We are somewhere on the west coast of the Antarctic peninsula. We will cruise around the various islands and through channels off the peninsula and view some of the research stations. Lots of whales, penguins, seals, and ice . . . After more scenic cruising we sailed north from Antarctica and stopped to view Elephant Island just north of the peninsula. This is where Ernest Shackleton's crew stayed, circa 1915, while he and two others sailed a lifeboat about 800 miles east to South Georgia Island, then hiked over the mountains to the whaling station on the far side, eventually, after several attempts, returning to Elephant Island to pick up his crew. I thought it would be just a pimple of a rock, but in fact it is quite large with several large mountains and lots of snow and glaciers.

Antarctica; January 30: Sailed north just east of the Falkland Islands. The east island can be viewed on the port side at a distance of about four miles . . .

Buenos Aires, Argentina; February 2 and 3: Arrived here this morning at about nine, after spending the night progressing slowly up the river. Apparently you have to follow the marked channel carefully or the river becomes too shallow. Buenos Aires is roughly 100 miles from the coast. The river is very wide (almost 100k at the mouth) and muddy. The main indication that you are on a river and not just in a bay is the color of the water . . . I will charge my chair for an hour and then take a little cruise around the city if I can manage to get out of the port area.

We are now waiting for another ship to pass because the river channel is not wide enough for two ships; we must anchor and wait for three hours even though the estuary is several kilometers wide, it is only deep enough in a marked channel that is wide enough for one ship.

When we finally get moving we will head out into the Atlantic for a seven-day crossing to Africa. Motion pills are at the ready.

At sea; February 4: The sea is as calm as a mill-pond today, and it's sunny. This is the first day of a seven-day crossing of the

Atlantic Ocean. Today is laundry day; I think I'll try to find a laundry room a little more accessible than the one I used last week. The laundry room doors are not quite wide enough, and I have a heck of a time entering . . . No luck, I don't think the ship's designers figured wheelchair people would be doing their own laundry. I'll just have to contend.

At sea; February 5, 6, 7: Again, very calm seas, sunny, just a few big rollers making things a bit interesting. The curvature of the earth is quite obvious when I pan around the horizon with no land in sight. A few ships pass from time to time, something I did not notice at all on the Pacific side . . . there are some sinister clouds on the horizon.

I am refining my dictation program today. When you do not use it much, it is very frustrating because it does not recognize my beautiful voice and flawless enunciation, and consequently I make a lot of annoying mistakes.

At sea; Monday, February 7: We are about halfway across the Atlantic. We have about three more days to go before reaching Africa. Getting some fairly rough seas today although nothing I can't handle . . . I hope to go on a tour of the bridge today, I haven't determined whether or not I can get on the bridge with a wheelchair, but I will find out this afternoon.

175

.   .   .

DAVE'S CRUISE log ends there. It was the longest and most personal correspondence he'd ever written. He does not mention the afternoon he spent in a doctor's office in Buenos

Aires having his mole removed. His wheelchair would not fit through the door into the doctor's office, so the surgery was performed in the waiting room. The mole was sent for biopsy, and the Argentinean doctor would send the results to the *Rotterdam*. Ten days after the surgery, Dave wrote to me: "Well, I haven't received any information on 'the thing' yet. I guess no news is good news. We are just leaving Cape Town, headed for Durban, South Africa."

My phone rang, early on Monday morning. Too early. It was a connection through which it seemed I could hear the crashing of waves.

"Marian, this is Dave." His voice was small, not just distant.

"Hi, Dave. Where are you?"

"Oh, just off the coast of Madagascar."

"What's up?" Calmly, my heart already in my throat.

"The report on the mole just came through. The doctor in Buenos Aires faxed it to the infirmary."

There was a crackling pause.

"He says it's a malignant melanoma."

Fear flooded my skin from within. I tightened my mouth so I would not cry.

"Oh, Dave—" I heard only silence over the vast distance between Toronto and the coast of Madagascar.

"The ship's doctor thinks I should come home right away..."

"We'll get through this. I'm going to call that nurse whose letters I mailed, was it Lorraine?"

Across the Holland America firewall, nurse Lorraine and I began a brisk correspondence. She faxed me the pathology report so that I could consult doctors in Toronto. The report was in Spanish. What, exactly, is melanoma, and how serious was his, and what was the process? I called everyone I knew in Toronto with medical connections. Did it make sense to get another biopsy in Mombasa or Tokyo or Hong Kong? If I could not get Dave appointments in Toronto for a month or so, should he stay on the ship? Lorraine and I exchanged e-mails, and then Lorraine talked to Dave. "Lorraine: I'm sure you're able to give him some calming assurance; one of the effects of MS on Dave is a tendency to panic, and when he is panicky he does not function well . . . " It was almost impossible for me to reach Dave by phone for some reason, and when I did he was calm, but his voice was flat, and I knew he was terrified. The *Rotterdam*'s next port of call with an international airport was Mombasa, Kenya, where Dave could connect through Nairobi to Paris and then to Canada. There were disagreements with the medical insurance company about whether or not this was an emergency; they would charge Dave more than US$14,000 for a medical attendant to fly with him. Lorraine and I decided he did not need one, as long as he had people to help him at airports and an indwelling catheter. "Dave: don't get too panicky or depressed . . . Don't stop taking your medication until you know what the arrangements are. Don't stop drinking. So, so sorry this happened, but we can deal with it."

The combination of MS and melanoma, with the ener-
vating effect radiation or chemotherapy would have, encouraged doctors in Toronto to treat Dave's situation as a matter
of urgency. He would be able to see a plastic surgeon within
24 hours of his arrival home and the melanoma specialist
within a week of his return to Canada. The samples were
sent from Buenos Aires to Toronto. A friend in the adventure travel business offered to provide someone in Paris to
meet Dave and transfer him to his next flight. Lorraine and I
worked out details:

"Can HAL expedite the paperwork for getting into and
out of Kenya? As you know, Dave cannot write... Also,
should I be making arrangements with a home care nurse to
have the catheter removed when he gets home?"

"The indwelling catheter should be no problem for him.
We'll get him a leg bag that is discreet and easily emptied. As
far as removing it, all you have to do is cut the valve, the bal-
loon will deflate and it slips out just like his regular one... "

"Lorraine, can Air France be given advance notice regard-
ing Dave's needs: like not being able to move on the plane
once he is seated, needing help cutting food and with landing forms. Oh, and tell him to drink more water than wine
on the flight, which could be a challenge on Air France,
and that I will be there in Toronto; I may not be able to get
through to the gate, but I will be right outside customs, as
close as I can get!"

"Dave, try to get as much sleep and rest as possible, take
deep breaths; drink water, stay calm. And again, women of

Holland America infirmary and beyond, thank you so, so much. We will get through this."

I don't know how he managed or who helped him to pack up his things, but he disembarked at Mombasa. His hospital bed and reclining chair continued on the ship to the Far East, across the Pacific, and were finally offloaded by Sara in Los Angeles.

. . .

Tuesday, February 22, 2000

Dear Lorraine, it is now Tuesday evening, and Dave is safely home. As you said, he is very resilient, and he was in remarkable shape after a 36-hour journey that included being lifted off a plane down steep steps by four men in Nairobi, sitting for 12 hours without moving on a sofa in Nairobi, going to a clinic in the Paris airport, and then to an airport hotel (courtesy Air France, who were helpful everywhere), where he slept for two hours, and then enduring an hour of mechanical problems in Toronto airport with his wheelchair (disconnected the wrong way on plane).

He must have been in very good health before he started the trip home, and he certainly has a very great sense of accomplishment about his trip thus far. He is surprisingly calm and knows that he did the right thing in coming home to deal with this.

Thank you from both of us. With any luck (I hope you agree!) he will be back on the MS *Rotterdam* next year. Warm regards, and enjoy the remainder of your millennium cruise.

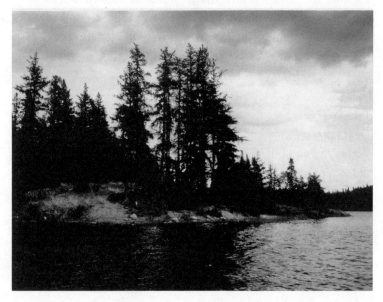

Dave's island, Lake Beaverhouse

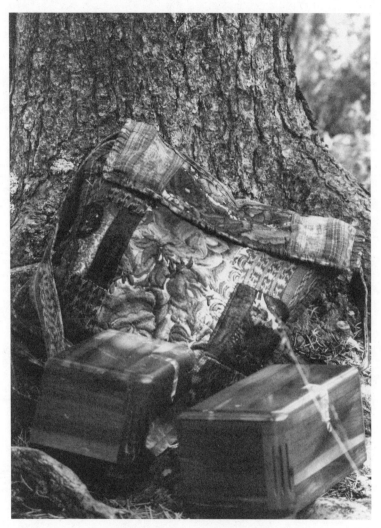

The cedar boxes and tapestry bag

5

THE

SHADOW-

STALKER

WE are on the island for about three hours. We wander severally down to the shore or back into the bush. It has been a dry summer, and some of the foliage looks burnt. The lake is eerily silent. We can see only one boat, that of the Beaverhouse band member, trolling along the shore down by the dam.

I stand for several moments beside Lorne, who is staring into the water. He tells me he used to think about Dave and himself as the characters in Earle Birney's poem "David"— two young men in their prime, who hike, climb, and camp in the mountains out west, as Dave and Lorne did in the years they both lived on Vancouver Island. It is a poem about youthful exuberance and deep, connected friendship, and the bliss of doing things together in the wilderness, "because we had joy in our lengthening coltish muscles, and because mountains were there for David to see over."

The poem ends in tragedy. David is impaled on a jutting ledge of rock after a fall, and he begs his friend to release him to the canyon far below—"you know I'd do it for you . . . ." Lorne (like the poet) stops here; he cannot bring himself to describe what happens next in the poem. He says only, "I often used to wonder if something like that might happen, Dave asking me to, uhm, help him . . . you know?"

"To die?" I say, with my hand on his arm, "I think probably not." I too had had variations on this scenario but could never see it, finish it.

About six weeks after Dave was diagnosed with melanoma, he was in his wheelchair walking Dobie along the lakefront, as he did without fail every day for four years. It was late March. Even in the worst weather he rarely wore socks and shoes, as it was too difficult for him to put them on and take them off. So he would have been wearing his backless leather slippers, sweatpants, his old red ski jacket with rope burns on it, and a cap. To walk Dobie, he had an expandable leash either looped over the handle of his wheelchair or held in his otherwise useless left hand. He used his right hand to maneuver the joystick on the chair.

His walk took him down a pathway lined with pines to a concrete sidewalk that ran along the lake. This sidewalk was in considerable disrepair, in places running right above the lake with no railing between the edge and deep water, about ten feet below. In a few places, large, round concrete bollards once planted with annuals had become filled with weeds, broken glass, and flowers gone to seed. They were joined by linked chain, about knee height, with no discernible purpose. Dobie, with his usual exuberance, pulled Dave into a left turn, alongside the bollards.

Dave's joystick suddenly jammed, and the wheelchair started to lurch and spin. It made a ninety-degree turn and headed swiftly, directly, toward the lake. It ran Dave right into one of the linked chains and then sat there whirring like a car spinning its wheels on ice. Dobie's leash and Dave's feet were also tangled in the chain.

There was a man on the sidewalk, who rescued them. If it had not been for that short piece of chain, Dobie on the leash and Dave in the chair would have gone straight over the edge and down ten feet into about twenty feet of frigid gray water.

Dave told me about this episode in his matter-of-fact manner a few weeks after it happened. I said, "Let's say you had gone over and no one was there, what we would have thought . . . " He grunted, noncommittal. "All I could think about," he said, "was the length of Dobie's leash, and the relative depth of the water. And I was worried because, according to my calculations, if the wheelchair was on the bottom of the lake, the leash would not be long enough to allow Dobie to swim to the surface."

My mind goes to this image now, but I don't share it with Lorne. I think Dave would never have killed himself. But I thought he might discuss the possibility with me when the lingering degradation of his body around his mind became unbearable.

At three o'clock, the sun is on its downward arc and the air is slightly cooler. I ask Jon to open the champagne. We collect the little cedar boxes, glasses, and camera, and we walk, single file and silent, along the faint trail through the bush to the point.

The sky is a pale ebbing blue of late summer, and the cumulus clouds are beginning to build above the orderly fringe of spruce and jack pine that march around the horizon at the far end of the lake. There is by now a steady breeze, brushing little waves across the rocky shore of the point.

We stand in an awkward clump facing the water. The two cedar boxes are side by side on a rock at my feet. Jon pours us each a glass of champagne. We don't know quite what to do or say. This is a family of performers and writers, people never at a loss for words. We are all mostly silent. Suki and Jon record. Gideon makes a toast, strong and simple words I cannot recall. Jon says something. I can say nothing, except that he was a brave man.

Not in a million years could I say what I want to say about my little brother, Davy. He emphatically did not believe in God, and he had his reasons for disbelief. A church service, pat words from a minister who never knew him . . . anything other than this return to this place of our childhood would have been wrong. Here are all the elements he loved: rock, water, stone, wood, the craftsmanship in the little boxes, his family. We only lack fire; he would have built and maintained the fire, as he always did. The ceremony is the journey, the rituals those of our childhood and our family.

186

August 2000

*I find it very hard to write about this, as I go through huge
waves of sadness, rage, anxiety, grim determination to manage, times of needing to sleep and sleep and sleep, after I
return home from spending time with Dave.*

   *It seems I can count the days when he was truly happy, on
his cruise, managing to do exactly as he had imagined, Dobie
content and pigging out at Bruce's, Dave's e-mails winging
silently from the ship. I could picture him so so clearly, at any
moment. And there were his funny photos, and his wry, terse
log, sent out with huge pride, because before he left he had
said he would achieve this—keep a cruise log—and he did.
So why, oh God, why, the melanoma halfway through?*

   *I hear his small scared voice on the telephone from the
MS* Rotterdam, *telling me about the biopsy results . . .*

. . .

BETWEEN THAT phone call and Dave's eventual appearance at the airport, wheeling himself through, looking
amazingly alert and happy, burdened with gifts and sou-
venirs after a thirty-hour flight from Mombasa, Kenya, I
plunged headfirst into the world of oncology and pathology. The specimens were sent from Buenos Aires to Toronto
and read again, in English, or something akin to English: a
malignant melanoma, nodular type, single atypical mela-
nocytes, focally noted; pagetoid spread not obvious, crust
present. Clark's level III/IV of invasion. Two days after his

return, I watched a plastic surgeon cut a section of flesh from his back like the slice of a fresh peach.

I went to Mexico for the month of March because I had a book deadline, and Suki's mother, Caroline, came from Vancouver to stay in my house and be "honorary sister" to Dave. There was, in any case, a pause between the biopsy and subsequent action. Caroline took notes and arranged for Wheel-Trans to take Dave to appointments and shuttled his X-rays from one hospital to another. She queried his diet in her firm Scottish way and found a caterer who would deliver good meals and even looked at a long-term care facility for MS patients that I had never had the courage to explore. I came back at the end of the month to a binder full of neatly written notes.

Sometime in April Dave and I made an evening emergency trip to Toronto Western for bowel problems; was it hemorrhoids or constipation? When we came back to his apartment after midnight I lost my temper, furious with his desultory hygiene. I poured Javex all over the bathroom floor and scrubbed his feet, and then I cried all the way home because I had yelled at him. I started delivering cooked prunes and apricots to the apartment for his breakfasts.

In May he had biopsies done on the lymph nodes on both sides of his body. (In an additional small curse, Dave's lymphatic system did not drain to just one side of his back like that of most people, but to both sides.) The biopsy results three weeks later showed a tumor and "melanin pigment" in his left lymph nodes. It was then 84 days until the surgery on August 4—although the oncologist, Dr. V—, called the

188

cancer an "aggressive melanoma," he seemed to think there was no urgency; the surgeon took his holidays. Dave chose quiet denial as his way of dealing with this long hiatus, but I insisted that we meet with the MS specialist because I wanted to know about the effects of anesthetic and surgery on someone with MS; I wanted the medical professionals to *see* Dave as someone with two possibly conflicting conditions. The MS specialist was very clear: MS will only take five or six years off your life. Melanoma might kill you.

There were two rocky weeks after the surgery. Dave had bad and good days at home; he was weak, unable to catheterize, and furious because he could not get physiotherapy immediately, and we all nervously awaited the pathology results. The tiny, cryptic report showed not a single trace of melanoma. We celebrated by spending one afternoon at a friend's cottage on Lake Simcoe, Sara and I and Dave and Dobie. We took a detour around Eastbourne, driving slowly down the road toward the summerhouse, and Dobie immediately started whimpering and wagging his tail and jumping up and down. He and Dave had not been there for two years. We had a day beside the lake that bore a faint resemblance to our happiest summerhouse days. As we drove back to the city at sunset Dave said, well, I guess that was my summer holiday.

. . .

Peaks and troughs, deeper troughs than peaks, floods of feelings that I can barely discern the meaning of, I guess simply because he is my brother. If he can barely cope, the same is true of me, but I have to be ruthless, organized, clear, strong, one step ahead at all times, running, planning, buying, fetching, carrying, paying bills, making claims, calling doctors' secretaries, sending letters, following up, following up, following up. Having Sara here for three weeks literally split the load, and I can scarcely imagine what I have done before on my own, and then she is gone again.

And this is just me, not even clocking Dave's agony, fear, rage, determination, stubbornness, resilience, his ability to recalibrate his daily schedule, over and over again doing what seemed impossible the first time. Is this rocking, rolling tumult how it is going to be from now on?

. . .

APPARENTLY. ON September 12 we visited the oncologist, who said there was close to zero percent chance, "not zero, but close," of the melanoma turning up anywhere else. Oh, we said, trying not be jubilant. Then he did a routine examination of Dave's armpits, moved his hands up onto his neck, and found a swollen lymph gland. He looked in his throat and found an infection, took a swab, and said it was likely the cause of the swollen gland, but, just in case, we should see him in three weeks.

Three long weeks later the redness was gone, the lump was not. But still the oncologist said maybe it wasn't melanoma; it seemed "smaller," it didn't "feel" the way melanoma does. The surgeon did a needle biopsy. He did not tell us (why?) but noted in his report that he could see the black specks of melanoma in the fluid he took out.

On October 13 another surgeon, Dr. B—, a short, tense, dour man, said that even if the cancer had not gone anywhere else, this new tumor meant Dave only had a 30 to 40 percent chance of surviving, or of recurrence, survival meaning achieving average life expectancy, which Dave did not have anyway, because of the MS. He recommended an aggressive surgery to remove all the lymph nodes on the left side. I asked the oncologist why he had not taken the biopsy when he first saw the lump, and he said because it was "plausible" that the sore throat was the cause. I came to dislike and distrust the word *plausible*.

Four days later Dave was in hospital for the surgery, preceded by a CT scan (in case there were any lesions elsewhere). The ward was the ear, nose, and throat (ENT) and head and neck ward, an unnerving place populated by people with tracheotomies, who made thick, rattling noises when they breathed, and with a rule-bound nurse who refused to catheterize Dave because the doctor had neglected to order it and she might lose her job. And doctors who never, never came. I paced in the corridor; after the CT scan I expected to hear from the surgeon who had promised me Dave would not be given bad news without me being present, but he just didn't come at all. His intern claimed to know nothing. The anesthetist said he was told the major surgery was going ahead, so we assumed, hurrah, the CT scan must be clear. But I overheard the desk nurse on the phone asking the resident about an ultrasound that had been ordered for Dave. I hovered by the desk. The assisting surgeon called in from home, was told by the nurse I was there, and he obviously said he would not speak to me because she muttered, but she is *right here,* so he could not refuse. When I got on the phone he turned down his sound system and said, there are "reasons to believe" there are lesions.

Dr. B— called me after the ultrasound the next morning. I was in the middle of a short-term communications contract with City Hall, in my cubicle, with breathing, invisible bodies on either side. Open-plan offices are bad places to receive bad news.

There were three "lesions," he said, enunciating clearly. The melanoma had "metastasized"; there were tiny tumors in his liver, in both lobes. I don't know why we have to use their language, but we do. There was no point in doing extensive lymph node surgery, as planned, he explained patiently. A focused procedure to remove the lump would be performed around noon.

The melanoma had jumped ship. Taken an invidious, invisible ride through Dave's bloodstream (where it leaves no trace) and set up a staging post in his liver.

I agreed to meet the surgeon in the pre-op room, to be there when he told Dave. I called Sara in Los Angeles, trying to be discreet, swallowing sobs. Sweet, pregnant Jodie in the cubicle next to mine silently handed me a box of Kleenex along the window ledge.

I met Dave in ultrasound and walked beside his stretcher down to pre-op; we did not discuss why I was there, but I am sure my eyes betrayed me. The surgeon came and told Dave the news and then left us to prepare for the now much smaller surgery.

I could do nothing except pat his hand, motionless on his green hospital gown. Neither of us cried in front of the other. Dave said, "Well, Dad always said I was a hypochondriac. I guess I showed him."

In the middle of the night after his surgery, Dave broke out in a screaming, swearing rage when a nurse refused to help him relieve a fiercely itchy arm he was too weak to scratch. Do it yourself, she said from behind the game on her computer. The next morning she said she had no idea he had MS.

FROM MY letter that day to Dr. V—:

.   .   .

Thank you for your careful and full report to Dave and me this morning. I just want to make sure that we got everything right. Our understanding is that you are going to:

1. order an MRI for Dave, after checking with the MS Clinic at St. Mike's so that his MS can be assessed at the same time.

2. order a CT scan in six weeks time. Changes to tumors showing at that point would indicate if liver surgery is an option, and we do understand that is unlikely, given the location of the tumors in separate lobes.

3. discuss with Sunnybrook the likelihood of Dave's eligibility for biological therapy, knowing he would have to take a genetic code blood test.

4. discuss with Dr. Flaherty in Detroit the likelihood of Dave's eligibility for their biochemo/interferon/IL-2 program while acknowledging that it is unlikely that Dave would be a good

candidate. (The therapy itself sounds grueling and the logistics in Dave's case are daunting.)

5. look into the option of standard chemo with added components; again, it is unlikely this treatment would yield a health benefit in Dave's case.

Dr. V—, I want to reiterate what I said this morning: I would never want or expect you to tell me something that I would keep from Dave. I was trying to catch you before you left the ward and also not to ask a confidential question in front of the orderly. I was upset that you thought otherwise . . .

That is not how our family works. In many cases it is quite the opposite; I deliberately do NOT make eye contact with doctors, so they will be forced to speak directly to Dave. People, even doctors, do not always treat a person in a wheelchair as someone with full mental capacity. This disrespect happens more frequently than you might think and so I am pleased that you respect Dave's intelligence. And as far as complex statistical information is concerned, as an engineer Dave is far better at processing stats than I am!

Thank you for your good and thoughtful care of my brother . . .

.   .   .

How Dave feels: impossible to tell, although he seems not angry, not depressed, almost reflective; is there some kind of relief and if so why?

He is weaker than he was six months ago, although it is genuinely impossible to say for sure, because events like surgery are hard on him and confuse the overall picture, and because I don't want him to be worse. But he does have to call the Participation guys every night to help him into bed. He seems not to be eating a great deal, only a yogurt at night, usually a decent meal at lunch and either the prune and yogurt breakfast or a pastry/coffee one. He will always eat if I bring a meal. He has lost weight, he says thirty pounds in the past three years, but this weight looks better on him and makes his mobility easier. His voice is soft. He could not stab the stupid Portuguese takeout potatoes last night; I think his right arm is weakening. He said at dinner—pensively— maybe laser surgery would work. I don't know what to think about his frame of mind.

He does not know about the letter from Holland America, detailing why they will not let him go again on a cruise without an attendant. They said he was a burden on staff. He remembers his trip with great pride in his accomplishment. He says he only needed help once, getting into bed. The truth is probably somewhere between his and theirs. He would not remember, willfully or otherwise, myriad small interventions. He would be treated with prejudice by some staff, who might tolerate extremely bad behavior from afflu-

ent, able-bodied passengers, but see every small need of a disabled person as extra work. Talk of resuming the cruise subsided in November.

How I feel: at first, crying hard, then exhausted, then cheerful, calm, organized, in control and not especially tense. Not at all sociable, although the night after his surgery I felt great pain and wanted a warm kind man to hold onto, so I called two good male friends and at least had the comfort of their voices. I do feel good about how we as a family work together on all this, how we support and laugh and care and trust. I feel really good about that.

. . .

WE WAITED. Every Sunday now we did a long outing together, me on my bike, Dave in his chair with Dobie trotting alongside. One crisp fall day we went down to the pier and boarded an old sailing ship that toured the harbor. The sky was a deep blue, gulls perched rakishly on bollards; the air was fresh, leaves golden on the islands. We sat in blissful silence under the snapping white canvas and watched young people as graceful as dancers run the boat.

The scan at the end of November showed no growth, and the MRI was clean. It seemed that we might cautiously resume a normal life. The MRI sat on Dave's desk like any other CD. We looked at it several times on his computer; we could see cutaways of his head, like slices of an apple or onion, the eyes poking outward like tubers, all the way down into the brain stem, where there was some white blotching; perhaps this was the MS, we said, but we had no idea how to interpret these images. We were told almost incidentally that the MS was only in his spinal cord, not in his brain.

Christmas. Dave and I and Dobie had a gloomy little morning together at my house. The weather into the new year was terrible. Dave had sharp pains in his shoulder and back and saw a rheumatologist, who diagnosed frozen shoulder and gave him a cortisone shot, which caused him subsequent great pain and no relief.

The winter dragged on. His deep-seated routines slowed and were shrunk by his increasing weakness. Up early, helped into his wheelchair, first priority downstairs with Dobie for a quick pee, bare feet shoved into the shabby backless slippers even on the coldest days. (He had not been able to put on socks for almost four years.) Then into his bathroom with a catheter from the microwave; catheter back into the microwave. Feed Dobie. Coffee, set up the day before by the Participation guys, some form of breakfast, muffin or sweet Danish or bran cereal; for a while he religiously ate the yogurt and prunes/apricots I cooked for him. The radio, CBC One, was always on in the morning. Into his chair, with his coffee and the paper; he switched back and forth from the *Globe* to the *Star;* he read what he could lift, or hold, pausing to rest, dozing as time shortened. The list of things on the fridge for the Participation guys to do grew longer.

I visited him with dread, with determination, with good things to eat, with bones for Dobie. Check the mail downstairs, throw out the junk. Bring the remainder up to him, opening some on the way, slow to realize I needed to open everything, only doing so in the last few months. Slow to realize I either had to forge his signature or help him do it. He was so determinedly independent that often I did not know the full extent of his helplessness; the Mom in him. Early on I would have announced myself on the intercom, but not for quite a while. I had keys. I always knocked and then opened the door and shouted a greeting; Dobie would bound over, grinning, keening in his weird way, tail whirring, nails clattering as he danced up and down. Dobie never lost this ridiculous eagerness to greet people. Put things down in the kitchen. Mostly, Dave was in his recliner, the top of his frizzy head visible, the TV on. For how many years did he tape Letterman every night and watch it the next day?

This winter he was virtually a prisoner of his chair, his TV, his catheter. He was getting physiotherapy and was irritated by the prickly ultrasound machine. He was helped more and more by the Participation attendants, with dressing, getting in and out of bed and wheelchair and chair, still managing the catheter, but finding the simple act of pulling his pants down and up very hard. I bought him three new pairs of pants and had the flies Velcroed. He was sharply aware of the difference between his mobility now and that of a year ago, on the ship. I imagine he thought of that difference every single day.

On March 9 Dr. V— called me at home with results of a CT scan ten days before. The 4-cm lesion had grown to 5.8 cm; the two smaller ones had also grown, and there were two additional very tiny ones. He recommended a low-toxicity chemotherapy, two treatments only, to try to shrink the lesions to half their size. And if the chemo did not work? He would not recommend any further treatments.

I took leftover stew and some movies on DVD to Dave. He was quiet, dozing off during a movie. I stroked his hair. I looked into his eyes and saw the pain and fear there. I felt that we were on a long, slow slope toward death.

. . .

The melanoma is a fretful, sleeping monster, a Grendel in the cave who occasionally rolls over, spreads out, wreaks damage and then slumbers again. "The shadow-stalker, stealthy and swift..."

The sorrow sits on my heart like a pillow, and I can do nothing.

. . .

THERE WAS no heart in this spring, but we took each day as it came, as if the days would always come. We planned a large cottage party for Sara's fiftieth birthday in early August, and I once again went looking for a wheelchair-accessible cottage so that we could take Dave for a summer holiday at the same time. On the Internet, I found a horrible little place on a small lake near Dorset, with two bedrooms, bunk beds in one, a hole in the bathroom floor for the shower drain. I drove three hours north and trudged in through thigh-high snow and took photos and imagined guests pitching tents in the woods and decided it would be fine. I booked it and with Dave made plans for this event. At the same time, he and I made financial, legal, and power-of-attorney adjustments, which suggested we had a different time frame in mind. He did one session only of chemotherapy, which brought another regime of drugs into play. We went out one evening, to a hockey game at the Air Canada Centre, and it was pleasant enough that he could wheel home afterward; I trailed him in my car like a spy and honked and waved when he was close to the co-op.

But we never spoke of death. He became thinner. He had symptoms and flickering pains everywhere. I have a searing memory of him, one late spring evening, curled toward the wall on his bed, sobbing, skin white but raw and red in places, tended gently by Rita with tears in her eyes while I held his hand.

In mid-May, we learned that the pain in his shoulder was also caused by an invasion of melanoma, three bony mass lesions in the glenoid fossa and shaft of the left humerus. He began a course of radiation. The effort of getting to and from the hospital—booking WheelTrans by phone, waiting for the ride, missing his ride home again because the radiation technicians got backed up, trying to rebook and waiting again or slowly, slowly wheeling himself home—became almost impossible. I tried to get him to use a wheelchair-accessible taxi service I had set up for him, but he rarely would. He forgot, or it was too much trouble or too expensive.

In early June, Grendel—"the dark death-shadow who lurked and swooped in the long nights on the misty moors"— struck again. The pathology reports showed lesions in his lung, breast, spine, spleen, adrenal gland, small bowel, and both kidneys. There was also a black spot on his face, and tumors we could feel on the back of his head but did not tell him about.

Dr. V— and I spoke at seven one morning on the phone about these reports. I, of course, asked, how long? He suggested Dave had between three and six months to live. When Dave and I discussed this report, he did not ask me how long and I did not tell him.

And still, we did not speak of death. Neither of us cried. The time I was least successful at self-control was the day we went to see Dr. T— the radiologist, a week after his final CT scan. Dave's eyes were bleak in a face now gaunt and white. He could scarcely sit on the foam cushion on his wheelchair. He ate only a third of a hot dog. We had a brief, sad conversation with little Dr. T—, who was the first doctor to talk directly with Dave about his prognosis, who said gently there was no point in radiation therapy, who offered only some ways of dealing with the dry and bitter-tasting mouth. Dr. T— gave me the scan results, which I folded and put into my purse and did not read until many hours later. Dave silently waited for WheelTrans, no longer able to wheel himself home.

Our mother's mother was a Bowers, one of four sisters. Whenever anyone in our family shows a tendency to cry, they are said to be "Oh, just like the Bowers girls. You cry like a Bowers girl." This was why Mom wore sunglasses. I too am said to cry like a Bowers girl. I hardly ever cried in front of Dave. Night after night when he was clearly exhausted or about to embark on one of his catheter nightmares, or in one already, I would say *Good night, Dave, take care, see you tomorrow, call you in the morning. Okay, Mare, thanks, goodnight...* and I would hear the apartment door close behind me and his keening would flow over into the corridor. My reserve would immediately break. I wanted to sag against his door and rage and howl. But I would force myself to walk to the elevator blinded by tears.

THERE IS a calm and secret garden in the snarled bureaucracy and erratic delivery standards of Ontario home care. It
is called palliative care, and it is home care as you imagine
it should be, just as the standard of nursing in a chemotherapy unit is the compassionate, hands-on, proactive nursing
of the past. In mid-June, my family entered the palliative
care garden. Because I had been through the deaths of two
close friends in the previous two years, I knew without hesitation that was the right move. Dave agreed to it, even as
we did not talk about the fact that he was dying, except to
acknowledge, wordlessly, the oncologist's prognosis. The
words that were his own epitaph he did not speak to me but
on the phone to his ex-wife, Kathy, in British Columbia; he
said, "I don't think I'm going to be around much longer."

But a cradle of care was built unobtrusively around him.
No, it was not unobtrusive; there was an influx of equipment: special mattresses, two different Hoyer lifts for transfers, spongelike Rojo cushions, a better hospital bed, a bath
chair. There were nurses who came regularly to visit and an
attentive young occupational therapist who wrote letters on
Dave's behalf after a detailed needs assessment. There was
a care manual and phone numbers that could be used and
would be answered twenty-four hours a day. And there was
Dr. David Ouchterlony.

In Kirkland Lake as children, we participated in the
Kiwanis Music Festival every spring, playing piano or singing solos or in choirs. The adjudicators always came from
southern Ontario, and the adjudicator I remember most
clearly was Dr. David Ouchterlony, a very tall man with a

long, lugubrious face and a wit that charmed ten-year-olds as well as their parents. He was the organist at Timothy Eaton Memorial Church in Toronto, which for some reason gave him additional authority. Now his son, David Ouchterlony of the Temmy Latner Palliative Care Centre at Mount Sinai Hospital, was to be Dave's doctor. He was also very tall with a long face and gentle wit. He had practiced medicine in northern Ontario, so he understood us, especially Dave, in some way I cannot explain, and in a further connection, he had once lived on Lake Simcoe in the very house that we had owned and called the summerhouse.

I was not there when Dr. Ouchterlony first came to Dave's apartment for a long and quiet consultation. Whatever transpired between them cleared the air of fear and anxiety. Dave accepted that he needed an indwelling catheter. This acknowledgment was both a source of considerable ease and a symbolic loss of power. That day, said my daughter, Katherine (who had come from Vancouver to help look after Dave for two weeks), Dave yielded to death.

For me, the presence of Dr. Ouchterlony meant that, for the first time, someone else was in charge. I had not felt that confidence with any other medical practitioner in the past ten years.

203

But when the palliative care nurse in a rush of goodwill suggested to Dave that instead of enduring the exquisitely painful transfer of his fragile bones from bed to wheelchair to reclining chair, as many as ten times a day, he should move his bed into the living room, he said, "No thanks, I don't think so. That would look terrible. People would think

I really was on my deathbed." He had had a conversation, as he often did, with Kathy, who would be coming to visit him on Monday, July 16. He wanted everything to look proper for their first visit since he left Campbell River in 1992.

Sara came from Los Angeles, planning to be in Toronto for July and August. Jonathan and Suki came through Toronto on their way west and spent several days with us. One night we all had dinner at Dave's; he was too weak to eat much, but we had a splendid family meal and told stories and showed photographs. Later we helped him to his bed and stood in a circle around him and laughed and massaged his feet and fussed over his covers. And still no one spoke of death.

He could not feed himself, so we would spoon some yogurt or scrambled egg with salami, a childhood pleasure, into his mouth. Katherine made smoothies. I got him a cyclist's water bag to place on the tray over his bed at night so that he could drink just by biting the tube. I would put it in the fridge, with water and ice, and written instructions for the Participation guys to put it on his tray, in the twilight of his days, to suck on in the solitude of the night. We laughed about the irony of this use of a cyclist's piece of equipment. He did not like it much, because it tasted of plastic.

His routine with Dobie if we were not there became almost impossible: he could barely put on the leash and take it off or lift his hand to push the elevator button on his return; sometimes he just had to wait for someone to push it for him, and then he would wait for the Participation attendants to come to put him in his chair. Yet how many times, when I asked him if this routine was becoming too much, did he say no, it was fine, he could do it. Rita: *Don't say you are fine, because you are not.* His reluctance to acknowledge his need for help was the huge block in caring for him, a block I had to climb over and over again to get to the next level of intimacy with him. His way of fighting was to figure out everything on his own. Dave never referred to me as his "caregiver" and in truth I still loathe the word because of its bureaucratic subtext. I never wanted to be his caregiver, just his sister. But as his caregiver, I had to choose the battles, with him and on his behalf, that were worth fighting. He gradually allowed me to help him, but we never admitted how much or exactly what I did, and he refused to accept solutions that required the presence, assistance, support of others, or that were, in his mind, alternative. Only a geologist or mining engineer gets joy in picking and scratching away at some obdurate stone (a 10 on the Mohr hardness scale). Dave was an obdurate stone.

I think he was rarely happy and probably angry most of his life, at least in later years. He was alone, silent, proud, stubborn and would not give anything emotionally to anyone. His passivity about MS was especially frustrating. The pride, the inability to say thank you, miserliness—many of his traits preceded the disease, were recognizable in childhood. He could only use force of mind, concentration, will power, determination. Anything else he considered weakness. He could not look at or think about the big picture, the long term, the context—only the immediate problem. He had, after the November news of metastasis, some form of acceptance, a small measure of reflection, a flickering capacity for grace, an occasional moment of candor. He allowed, finally, a short course of massage and admitted it helped him. Dr. Ouchterlony was clear that he was not fighting his death; he accepted it, but he did not want to be given a time frame. But he gave no indication of knowing or of wanting to say anything. Did he know we loved him? Did he love us? How were we to know? Because he tried so hard to be undemanding, because he wrestled in such a fiercely solitary way with his misery, rarely complaining or asking for help?

One night Sara cut his hair very short, and he looked like a little boy. On a sunny afternoon early in July he and I and Dobie went for our regular walk along the lake. His long fingers could scarcely nudge the joystick to keep his wheelchair moving. He spoke in a harsh whisper, which I had to bend down to hear. We were not out for long.

Death came swiftly, on a Saturday afternoon. It was the day of the Molson Indy, which took place two blocks from Dave's building, and so the high-pitched, incessant, penetrating roar blended with the sound of the air conditioner in his apartment and the sound of the television and the sound of Dobie, panting in the heat. I had taken him home with me the night before and this afternoon would take him to the kennel, where he would stay until Monday, to be groomed before Kathy's arrival that day. Dave was frail, tired; he said, "I think we should get Dr. Ouchterlony to come on Monday, because I'm not getting any better." He asked me to water the hibiscus, with giant coral blooms, on his balcony. And to move the MedAlert bracelet and his watch as low as possible on his wrist so that it would take as little effort as possible to reach them. I left with Dobie just past noon to get to the kennel before it closed. A young Participation attendant saw him around one, when he was dozing. Sara was there by three and called me to come immediately.

Dave was gasping for breath, roaring, eyes rolling into his head, but he told us calmly what his blood pressure should be and how to convert centigrade into Fahrenheit as we took his temperature. The young palliative care doctor on call came and said he should go to Emergency. Within seven minutes, ambulance attendants, fire fighters, and police were in the apartment, because the doctor used the words "short of breath" when she called 911. She also told the paramedics, "He is in palliative," and when they shrouded him in orange and bundled him on the stretcher and put him in the ambulance, his living will was resting on his chest. Code palliative; do not initiate life-saving measures. I rode in the ambulance beside the driver, a powerful, calm goddess with tumbling red curly hair. We drove straight down the middle of oddly deserted streets. In the far distance, I could hear the roar of the Indy, and in the near distance I could hear the sound of a siren. It took me some time to realize that the siren was us.

"I don't think your brother is long for this world . . ."

We were in Emergency at St. Mike's; it was a serene night, few other patients, few people milling around, all the activity behind closed curtains. The ER doctor's gentle, simple words: I don't think your brother is long for this world. I remember, over and over, the sharp curve of Dave's cheekbone against mine as I murmured into his ear and the wetness of his cheek and the dryness of his hand in mine and his mouth turning away from the oxygen mask until I asked that it be removed, his breathing harsh and gasping, then quieting, then separating, with pieces of silence between breaths, and his eyes still, pupils enlarged by morphine, my hand stroking his hair so recently cropped by Sara, his ridiculous neck pillow on the bones of his shoulders.

I want to understand that curious mix of sorrow and soaring that I felt in the hour—although it seemed much, much shorter—leading to Dave's death. I was conscious of so many things: his breathing most of all, his physical aspect, the monitor (flickering, restless, distracting), the tubes, the discreet intervention of a nurse, then the doctor unhooking the paraphernalia, and then just the three of us: Sara's bowed head, the Kleenex boxes, the mingling of tears that flowed unchecked down all of our faces. The sound first of my voice and then of hers, a rush of the memories we knew would touch him most deeply, pouring from us both, like a litany, a jubilate: ... *the Coppermine... the summerhouse... Antarctica...*

But I was also aware of something like exhilaration as I witnessed his death, knowing that it was almost sweet, probably utterly without pain, as swift and graceful as his journey from the top of Whistler to the bottom, or the beat-ing-heart passage along the Vancouver Island coastline on his Sunday afternoon century cycles between his house on the sound and Courtenay. A compressed, graceful, rhyth-mic journey that we were privileged to watch, be part of, embrace with memories and tears and rare physical close-ness. And a dignity that he fought for and was often denied in his final several years, when he had to allow himself to be cared for, to be vulnerable, to be less than completely independent.

His breath: that this should mark the drama of his pass-ing; it was something he refused to pay attention to or work with in life, and yet he must have heard it and consciously used it on his silent journeys on his racing bike, on his skis. The gasping did not bother me as much as it did Sara, per-haps because it was regular, audible, the outward sign of life in his already almost immobile body. He was not in a coma. His breathing became slow, quieter, paced, it seemed, with silences, preparing to stop like a cooling engine. His mouth was open, but twice, distinctly, he brought his lips together and smiled that little grimacy grin that was so characteristi-cally him. And then all was still, so still, calm, peaceful. His tense, stiff body relaxed. It is ten past eight, the guardian angel said as she took his pulse and found none.

It was as good a death as it could have been, a vindi-cation of his past terrible year. As if someone finally had decided to give him a break. He would not have borne well a lingering, painful decline, the loss of his carefully held routines in his apartment with Dobie, a period in palliative care no matter how palliative. People said how shocking, how fast, how soon. But I knew with every fiber of me that it was the best possible death, for him, for anyone. And that we three were together, him, as always, always after we were no longer children, the tall, strong one in the middle, was a gift from somewhere, someone.

But so much knowledge and feeling lay unspoken between us. A month or so before his death: Dave, I said, we should talk about some things. You mean while I am still lucid? Yes. One night, as I bathed his rough, swollen feet, he said softly, I can remember every single moment of my cruise.

The night before he died, as I massaged his feet with a soothing cream, looking down at what I was doing, I asked: Is there anything you want to talk about, anything you are worried about? No, he said.

What do you think about as you lie here? Nothing, he said, very softly. Everything.

It is disconcerting to recall that he died at 8:10, and Sara and I were home by nine. But there were four extraordinarily intense hours leading to his death, and half an hour afterwards, and neither of us could see the reason to linger with his body, stiffening again. I don't think he would have wanted us to. This body was not who he was.

There was a sweetness in him when he was a child, a light in his eyes that he lost, somewhere along the way. In the days before his death on this day—July 14, 2001—the features of his face, above the bony, pain-wracked frame, were once again those of that little boy.

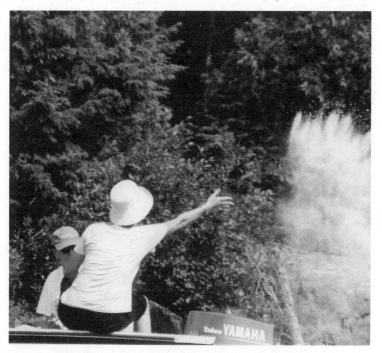

Sara throwing ashes at the mouth of the Sourdough

6

A SHADOW

I N

SHADOWLAND

WE open one of the little cedar boxes, and Sara and I each take a handful of the dense, chalky ash. It clings to our hands. We go to the water's edge and stretch our hands out over the water. The ash slips from our grasp, hangs briefly in a cloud, and then is whisked away by the wind, settling in a broad swathe on the black waters.

The children and Lorne do the same, and then we all take turns scooping out the ash and sending Dave's soul out over the waters of Lake Beaverhouse until the one box, at least, stands empty.

Katherine gives me one long, strong, fierce hug. Sara's children embrace her.

The light on the return journey is golden, warm on the rocks. Sara asks Lorne to make a turn around the mouth of the channel to Sourdough Lake so that she can throw some ashes there. Now the landscape plays out exactly as

Sara and I remember it, every cliff in its place, smaller now, or shrouded in trees. The children are content in the boats.

When we come to the narrow channel, we pause, daunted a little by what is now a brisk head wind and the current running against us. But as we consider our approach, the Beaverhouse band member in the boat, who has been discreetly close by all day, comes alongside us and then slowly leads us through.

Somewhere in the last portion of the river, I realize I am still wearing Dave's watch on my wrist. I stand and throw it into our wake.

And finally that night, after a blazing red and purple sunset, the rain comes—hard, strong, fierce, pouring from the heavens.

. . .

July 4, 2002
Bought cherries today, and thought of Dave, how he loved cherries. And pickerel, and melon, and how he hated green beans but liked broccoli, and how almost to the moment of death he could be cheered by something good to eat.

214

Wearing right now the blue linen shirt I wore that final day. Did his laundry that morning, threw bleach in to deal with soiled underwear and turned his briefs into tie-dye pieces, and there are bleach splashes on my shirt. We joked about this. We always joked. Sara and I craved his rare moments of lightness, humor, our wit. It was how we showed love, the only way. Oh we could tell that the family mattered to him, but he

could never tell us that, ever. As with Dad, we took our infor-
mation obliquely.

Forcing myself to write this evening about him, because
it is almost a year now, rounding into the final week lead-
ing to his death, and I still feel such sorrow, such pain that I
am unable to write anything. I have felt a great stone sitting
on my creative spirit. I cannot budge. I listen over and over
again to "Shadowland," the k.d. lang song that for years was
his lullaby in the CD *machine beside his bed.*

What surfaces...

The terrible clothes he wore, uncaring about stains and
dribbles, green T-shirts, baggy shorts or pants, no shoes
unless he was going out, and even in winter sometimes no
socks, because everything was so hard to do. Always, a ball
cap. He could not bear the heat of the sun.

Fear no more the heat of the sun...

Transfers. Stand, swivel, sit, stand, swivel, sit: transfers.
Everything was a transfer. Everything took forever and was
exquisitely calibrated: where his left hand went, the position
of his feet close to the chair, using only his right hand and
arm to bear weight. So, so, slow when he did it on his own,
and agonizing to watch and so often he made you watch,
refusing help, or only taking the kind of help that came as an
instruction from him. He insisted, way beyond truth, that he
was too heavy for us to manage; he had this idea of himself
as a big man.

Increasingly slight, skin on bones, hands graceful, his
eyes large in a handsome face. Lovely feet when they were

215

not scraped and bruised and calloused and torn by bashing into walls or on the foot rests of his chair or dirty from grazing the floor.

I am terrified of losing him.

. . .

IN THE six weeks after his death, I swam in eight bodies of water in Ontario and Michigan, conscious of immersing myself in pools of mourning. Each body of water had a particular significance: the waters north of Manitoulin Island, where he canoed as a camper; the three lakes (Crystal, Kenogami, Beaverhouse) around the town of Kirkland Lake, with intense childhood memories; Torch Lake in northern Michigan; the Ottawa River, where I walked on the shore with my best friend from childhood and talked to her mother, who was my mother's best friend and who also had MS; the little lake in the Kawarthas, where Dave had installed the beautiful cherry counter in our friend Frank's cottage; and again to Georgian Bay. I carried with me photographs of him, and I told, over and over again, the story of his death to people who knew our family, each time receiving a different form of consolation from the listener. I repeated this ritual without realizing what I was doing until the six weeks were over and it was September, that moment in any year when there is a return to the real world.

I still feel guilt, anger, resentment, flashes of emotion that shoot out in various directions, even though I know, absolutely clearly, I could not have saved Dave's life. I cannot think of Participation without anger. I hated their indifference, their erratic service, their helplessness, the stupidity of some, the slowness of others. Dave had a rough camaraderie with two or three of the good attendants, especially Bruce, who adored Dobie but who quit one day and left without saying goodbye to him, which hurt Dave obscurely. One attendant, less than two weeks before Dave died, stood over him in his wheelchair and threatened to withdraw services, telling Dave he would not transfer him anymore unless he got a transfer harness. (There was one, called a Hoyer lift, sitting for the longest time in a corner of the bedroom, but no one used it. The guys said Dave would not use it; he said they demanded training, or that they preferred not to, or ...)

I was terrified in the last nine months, alone with his pain, his weakness, his frustration, his helplessness. Sara and Katherine were three time zones away on the west coast. I didn't think anyone took seriously my fear, exhaustion, helplessness. If I had known how long, I could have moved in with him toward the end, slept on the pullout couch. I imagined doing these things, but much later—weeks, months, whatever time period the doctors predicted, which was weeks, months longer than he actually had. I could have been there all day the day he died, instead of leaving him alone for several hours. I could have tried harder to fix the TV before leaving that day with Dobie to get to the kennel before it closed.

I fret because I do not know what he thought or felt about death as it drew over him like the shadow of a cloud. Because I never once heard him say, "I love you." And because I, I, could scarcely say those words to him, only under cover of a laugh and a pat on his back, only tossed over my shoulder as I walked out his door.

Just once—when Sara and I had bullied our way into the pre-op room and we were all laughing about being rottweilers and about how horrible we looked in green hospital gowns and paper hats—he said with a grin, "Whatever you do, don't mess with my sisters."

IN MY dream I am tired. I go up for an afternoon nap to the room in the Dobie house that was sometimes the spare room and sometimes Sara's room. I am sitting on the bed with the carved, Eastlake headboard, the one I once scratched with a bobby pin. People keep bursting in and out of the room and dogs as well. Dobie is there. I shoo everyone else out, but Dobie stays, his big, eager yellow Lab face resting on the side of the bed, brown eyes alert, tail wagging. I start to talk to him, and he responds. I ask him if he remembers Dave, and he isn't sure. I say, do you remember who you were with before you went to live with Katherine's dad? Dobie is vague, grinning (he is still very much a dog, but he speaks like Dave in this dream).

Then a hologram (like the ones in the film *Minority Report*, home movies projected on glass) starts to form in the bedroom wall. A summer scene moves right out of the red-rosebud wallpaper; there's a lake, big maples in sunlight, like the summerhouse lawn, and then a figure moves out of the wall. It is Dave; he is slim, walking, smiling as in one of the pictures in the photo album. This hologram is warmly colored, very real, and Dobie is grinning his Lab grin and wagging his tail furiously.

I ask Dobie again if he remembers Dave, and he almost does, but it is clearly not a strong memory. Then Dave comes to stand beside the bed, and he asks if Dobie remembers him. Sara is also there, and we both know the answer. I tell Dave that Dobie does remember him.

DAVE'S DANCE with melanoma was preceded and contained by the long, slow seduction and possession of his body by multiple sclerosis. For as long as Dave was ill, or from the time of his formal diagnosis with MS, ten years before his death, we struggled to understand this infuriating, enigmatic disease, as if understanding it would have helped at all. We knew one person with MS, the best friend of our mother, who was diagnosed in her early 40s and at 90 was still alive and surprisingly well in many respects, even though she was bound to wheelchair and indwelling catheter and an overnight oxygen tank, reliant on conscientious home care and a patient husband. But her mind and her skin were clear until her death. Her eyes sparkled.

Otherwise, what we knew came from what Dave experienced, what we observed, and what we read. There are countless descriptions of multiple sclerosis, which takes many forms. The heart of the matter is always an attack on the myelin that coats nerves, like insulation over wiring that enables the wires to remain connected and

219

conduct current, information between the brain and every-thing else in the body.

Dave's diagnosis was made early in 1992, with an MRI in Victoria. Between that diagnosis and his death, nothing happened to make Dave's MS symptoms better; there is no cure for MS, but some forms can be slowed down by inter-feron drugs like Betaseron. Dave was not a candidate for these treatments, because it was determined at that time that such drugs could only help people whose MS was the "attack/remission" pattern. Even if the drugs became avail-able to those with chronic progressive MS, at best they would only slow down the disintegration. There was no possibility of reversal; Dave would not have gotten better, but he might have not gotten worse. Most people with MS have the attack/remission form, and so, logically, most of the research and treatment experiments have been on that form.

The CD containing the MRI images of Dave's head and neck sat on Dave's desk until he died and since then has sat on mine. Occasionally, I would put it into my computer and look at it; what did I expect to understand? It was like a postage stamp collection from another planet: black and white squares with writing in a foreign language. Shapes that were maybe a skull, a gap for an ear or nose? Two bulg-ing protrusions that were surely his eyes . . . There was a curious sense in which this MRI was somehow a piece of Dave, and I wanted to understand it.

I took the disc to a neurosurgeon for translation. I could scarcely follow his explanation, which he thought was per-fectly clear, but it was still in a foreign language.

"I do not see in the cerebellum or cerebrum or brain stem any really large areas of demyolating plaque," he said. "Oh, there is one, here . . . "

"Where?" I asked, seeing only black, gray, and white masses, and sometimes bone is black and sometimes it is white.

"Right here," he said, pointing to a tiny spot in the middle of the image. "On the right side of the upper medulla, in the brain stem."

"Oh," I said, still seeing nothing. "And all this white stuff?" (Because I thought the white areas meant brain deterioration.)

"This flare shows quite a good distinction, and white shows up as black in an echo projection," he said.

"I see," said I, not seeing at all.

"There are no huge serious streaks of plaque," he said, flipping briskly through the images. "In fact, this isn't a typical picture of MS. It is not diffuse; it is very focal." He snapped from screen to screen. "This brain looks quite normal," he said. "There is no atrophy, no hydrocephalus, no mass, no deformity no . . . formations . . . no tumors."

221

He wondered if Dave had ever had anything like a stroke, telling me about Wallenberg Syndrome, which struck the same spot and resulted in swallowing and speech difficulties. No, I said. Not to my knowledge.

"Was his MS ever proven by a lumbar puncture?" he asked.

"Not to my knowledge," I said again, realizing that this MRI was the only evidence I had ever seen of Dave's MS.

"So, only there," I said. "Just there?"

We were looking at a spot, a curved pocket in the brain stem that would be smaller than a dime. The neurosurgeon turned off the machine and handed me back my brother's brain. "We are looking very retrospectively through a haze of imprecise history," he said gently. "And it only contributes to the mystery of it all."

THREE YEARS after Dave's Day, I returned to northern Ontario. I stayed in a little cabin on Beaver Lake, about five miles as the crow flies from where we scattered Dave's ashes on Lake Beaverhouse. Beaverhouse and Beaver lakes share some of the same swampland, reorganized by the same extended family of beavers no doubt, but they do not quite belong to the same chain of lakes. There were only two cabins on what I thought of as my lake, mine and that of Don from Larder Lake, who had built them both. Again it was August, a miserably cold month. It rained for days on end.

One day I went back up Lake Beaverhouse with Gaston, a friend of Don's.

Gaston was originally from St. Georges de Beauce, near the Quebec/Maine border, but he had been in northern Ontario since 1988; he loves it here, because of the hunting and fishing. He drives heavy equipment, but "I'm on the pogey, me"; he has been laid off twice in three years because, as he understands it, there's some "tax" the Americans pay Canada to inhibit lumber production. He had never worked underground; he worked only for the sawmills.

222

Gaston is tall, solidly built, with a high-sitting small pot belly; since he got laid off in April he had gained fifteen pounds. His girlfriend of 20 years is Carole, who works at the motel restaurant in Larder. He makes oblique jokes, with a straight face. He has a small mustache, thick white hair; he must be around 50. His English is clear but heavily accented and colloquial. Gaston hunts for moose—calf only, so he doesn't need a tag; he goes deer hunting south of North Bay some years. He hunts partridge but not ducks. In the winter he ice fishes on Larder Lake; in summer he also fishes, but he won't eat pike in the summer, "because of worms, eh, and the same is true of bass; only pickerel and lake trout are good in summer."

Gaston came out the lurchingly rough road to pick me up at the cottage, "to save the wear and tear on your car," and we stopped in Larder for his trailer and boat. He has a neat, small house, screened-in porch, a small garden. Gaston brought a small cooler with lots of water, toilet paper in a clear sack, life jackets. I had made sandwiches. We headed for the landing on Howard Lake.

It had been a rainy, cool spring and summer, and the roadside bush was bursting with color and sound. This northern Ontario landscape is rarely grand. It is a subtle mosaic built from myriad tiny elements: berries, flowers, chipmunks, warblers, hummingbirds, blue jays and whiskey jacks, kingfisher, loons and eagles, ravens and herons and dragonflies; it is familiar and pretty, even at its most modest. The wildflowers are close to spectacular: pink fireweed,

223

a lovely large mauve flower called Spotted Joe-Pye Weed, asters in several shades, yellow and white daisies, Queen Anne's lace, a bright mauve thistle, the occasional looming mustardy mullein, lots of a white pearl-button-like flower, intense yellow goldenrod.

The bush rolls almost imperceptibly from small black lake to a flickering marsh up to a thickly flowered roadside, then to really thick forest—rippling aspen, pale, leaning birch, the sharp silhouettes of individual pine and spruce trees. The startling outcrops of pink or rust or pale gray rock, and then another small black mirror of a lake, with a splattering of creamy water lilies, the cattails fringing the road, and high bush cranberry (white clusters turning blush), chokecherry, blueberry, wintergreen (red) berry, black snakeberry, raspberry, another rosy pink berry on a shrub I cannot name, mountain ash about to appear and the burgundy fur of sumac, and a burst here and there of maple already orange and red. Oh, and the lichen and moss, and blueberry bushes turning rosy red. Rosehips . . .

And the liveliness of the sky, day and night, the drama of clouds and wind in trees and on water. Northern lights, pale green beacons flickering on the northern horizon like some revealed city. The sky at three in the morning, bristling with stars.

None of this is tame, or tamed. It is just there, on long, long stretches of road (dirt, gravel, paved, sand, ribbed corduroy and blacktop and highway) joining desperate little towns, lined with small houses, once tarpaper, now vinyl, even lilac-colored vinyl. There are very few pretty towns in this part of the country; the towns are hardscrabble, utilitarian, temporary. This paradox of northernness remains something that those who leave the north long for at some level but cannot bear to fully experience. We crave, still, the beauty, smell, land, water, sounds, the symphony of seasonal change, but we are not able to embrace the dark side, the daily reality of life in the north, the look of these beaten-up towns and worn-down people with gray skin and shapeless clothes. The overcoat of small-mindedness, grounded in nothing more terrible than ignorance, the harsh side of that rough, crude humor that we certainly absorbed. These things attended our growing up here, and they shaped our shadow mother, from whose image our eyes still slide past.

But there was then and there is now a deep kindliness of people looking out for other people. A goodness and trust in small transactions and an irrepressible cheer and resilience. An ease between complete strangers, because we share a love of this bush.

It was a cool, mostly cloudy day, with some sun, pleasant for being in the boat, with no wind. Gaston and I headed down the river, toward Lake Beaverhouse. Again, I found this body of water magical, pleasing in a profound way. The water was much higher than it was three years ago; there was very little dried-up or dead bush; everything was green, with lots of lush grasses and reeds along the shores where there had been none then.

When we got to the Indian land, we pulled the boat up to a rickety dock slung amongst the grasses along the shore. At the height of summer, there were a number of people in residence, smoke curled from a chimney, a dog ran up and down the foreshore, where rowboats and canoes were pulled up. The village was a row of small cabins, some very old log ones, other newer, vinyl clad, strung along a mown pasture, ringing the curved, grassy shore. Every house faced the water, a large bay containing several small islands that also bear houses. This community is the Beaverhouse First Nation; they have a band office in Kirkland Lake, but it is not a reserve; the application has been pending since 1974. One polite young native man, standing in front of his cabin, said, "The government still owns us, but we are fighting that."

The old white wooden church had been demolished, but it was being rebuilt. Five men were building the new church. It was almost where the old one was, but it was larger; it had an airiness about it and a height that would be pleasing. It was to be lined with pine, but the outside would be vinyl. The old one had been sitting on rotten foundations; the materials were salvaged by the community, used in building on this land.

I wandered back into the cemetery, where I saw that there had been two burials already that year. There were almost a hundred graves in a clearing in a grove of aspen, balsam, and mountain ash and spruce. The graves were close together, in rows, some with mounded earth. Many of the wooden markers have rotted and broken and fallen. Two granite gravestones identified their occupants as privates in the Canadian Forest Corps. Other stones honored Mattias, the last traditional (hereditary) chief, and Alex Languef, my father's trapper friend, who was indeed buried here: 1911–1988.

Standing in front of the church beside a tiny old woman, I felt the sacred power of these waters. I doubt that either of us could have articulated what that quality is, but we shared the recognition.

Gaston and I continued down the lake. The channel this time was easily run, with only rocks at the entrance; we slipped over those burrowing deep in the dark water. We went right to the end of the lake, through the exquisite long channel with high cliffs on both sides plunging straight down into the water, past the island where we had Dave's ceremony.

At the far end of the lake there were two or three parked vehicles on shore and a pontoon boat, made of oilcans and pipe and old plywood, tethered to a sapling. We beached our boat just above the small rapids and walked along the corduroy and graveled road, up to the site of the abandoned Upper Beaverhouse mine. Two blue jays shot up out of the bush on either side of the road, like sentries. On the slight ridge to the south there was crude, extensive clear-cutting, which had rutted and scarred the landscape in an ugly, brutal way. (The young Beaverhouse man had warned us: "You won't recognize it." And it had obliterated their own trail, which was centuries old, the track that the people of Beaverhouse used to walk in the old days, from the lake to Dobie, maybe to the train station, and from there into town, meaning always Kirkland Lake.) Gaston wondered how this clear-cutting could happen when, as an individual resident, he was not permitted to cut a single tree beside a road or a lake.

We found the old shaft, filled and fenced in, the broken chunks of some concrete structures, twists of rusted wire and pipe. We climbed down through thick blueberry patches. I sat, for the sheer pleasure of doing so, in the crunchy white lichen, surprisingly stiff to the touch, and stroked the deep, thick green moss. We clambered up to the large hill of waste rock and some drill core, overlooking the river. There were small plastic bags of drill sample, ground-up rock, bags labeled, each one a distinct color, strewn around the piles of rock. Gaston poured out five bags, and we looked at five heaps of ground rock: black, gray, greenish-yellow, brown, a chalky white, but we could not come to any conclusions. We were doing what all northerners do, looking for gold in someone else's detritus. Every chunk of rock that sparkled, or a distinct vein, we saw as a missed fortune.

The Misema River below us was black, wide, flowing in a large, easy curve from the two sets of rapids at the end of the road. There were some very large old spruce trees. We found extraordinarily beautiful chunks of rock, and I collected some to bring home in one of the sample bags. We saw a partridge and three garter snakes, one very long.

Gaston was chivalrous with toilet paper and water; he carried my bag of rocks, and he would happily have gone anywhere I wanted on the lake. He was clearly enjoying the day. Northerners have a complex relationship with the environment, or rather the bush. They know it well, are comfortable in small boats, walking with a gun, sitting in an ice hut in winter. They have the machines to get through it: snowmobiles, ATVs, small boats. There is considerable grace in a man launching a small boat, and everything is neat and to hand, and a young man can take his small son fishing at dusk in the summer in a trice. There is an unselfconscious watchfulness, attention to the sudden flurry and squawk of birds or the sharp trill of an irritated chipmunk or a slight movement in the underbrush beside the road. Mostly this attention is simply curiosity and delight, and at times it is the attention required of a hunter.

But northerners don't kill for the pleasure of killing; they hunt because they enjoy the game of hunting, and they like to eat game. One moose will feed a large family over winter. Everyone agrees that pickerel is a delicacy. People have a sense of living in a place where wildlife is abundant; they fully expect to see bear, moose, deer. They believe the animals know when it is hunting season. They believe they have the right to make a living from this landscape. Their relationship with it is not abstract—it is immediate and practical. While they are happy to have the jobs attached to resource exploitation (clear-cut lumbering, sawmills, treatment plants and pulp and paper mills, open-pit and underground mining and milling), they do not see themselves as exploitative or disrespectful of the land. Gaston had contempt for the ravages of clear-cutting and for those who left litter on the shore of Lake Beaverhouse. These were the things that Gaston and I and his friend Don talked about.

Just beside Dave's island, we cut the motor and sat in silence. We saw a young eagle flying overhead and then standing on a branch in one of the spruce trees, in that characteristic wide footballer's stance, head fierce, with the curled beak. We saw a family of ducks, a merganser daycare, and one kingfisher flying low above the water.

We made our way back to the landing at Howard's Lake. There were no other boats on Beaverhouse and just one at the end of Howard's Lake.

The pace of this day was easy, relaxed, unhurried— everything took as long as it took, and there was no sense of urgency or drama. It was a typical northern day in summer. I was back on Beaver Lake by six and went out in the kayak. I saw several young eagles and, finally, a bear, ambling along the shore, clambering up and down fallen trees, looking for grubs and bugs. It may have heard me or caught my scent at one point; it was standing still, ears up.

At dusk, Don and Gaston pulled up at my dock in their small outboard and presented me with a slab of filleted pickerel, its translucent white flesh still streaked with a trail of blood. I heard them giggling like schoolboys across the water as they putted away.

I kayaked again in the evening. It was still and silent, the lake an obsidian window reflecting the sky. The half moon was like a piece of polished cloud, left over from some party in the southern sky. A single trail of jet stream in the north and nothing else in the sky. A train passed slowly, and twenty minutes later I heard the whistle again over a great distance. I sometimes felt the movement of a fish beneath the boat as a deflected sound wave. The shoreline was a thick tapestry of several shades of green and white and gray, a few beautiful, tall aspens standing out in shape and thickness, thin jack pines and spruce trees competing for height, white poles of rotted birch trees still upright, imbedded in the thicket of brush, beaver detritus, and mossy shore.

From Don's cabin in the next bay, I heard Diamond, his springer spaniel, bark, just once, and the sound echoed. A familiar scene floated again into my mind.

Dave and I on the bike trail along the Toronto waterfront,
I see him motoring along very fast,
Dobie trotting along
Just in front of Dave's wheelchair.
I am cycling slowly behind,
It is a perfect fall afternoon.

Then Dave's image slowly,
Slowly,
Fades,
Like the Cheshire cat,
Moving into middle distance
Until he disappears altogether.

There is only Dobie,
Trotting along,
Coming to the fork in the path close to home.
Looking over his right shoulder at where Dave should be
To ask,
As he always did,
Which path are we taking today?

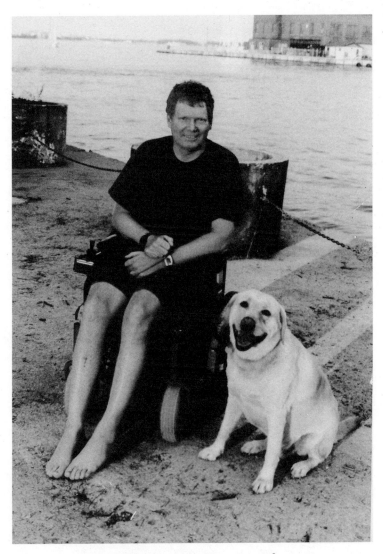

Dave and Dobie on the Toronto waterfront

PEOPLE sometimes ask: why did you want to write this book?

A male friend proudly told me this story: "Just before my knee surgery, I was told I'd be catheterized—for my comfort afterwards. When I demurred, I was told I'd have to talk to the surgeon. So when the orderly said, 'Get on this stretcher so I can take you to the operating room,' I said, 'No, thank you, I'd rather walk,' which I did. I wanted to be able to stand and look the surgeon in the eye for the discussion about the catheter. We agreed I wouldn't need it."

As I listened, I could only think: those simple choices (to be independent, be seen as an equal, be part of the decision-making process) were not available to my brother. First disabled people are dealt the blow of various forms of incapacity, and then they suffer the further indignities of discrimination, thoughtlessness, ignorance, debilitating bureaucracy, and even cruelty. The man in the wheelchair is invisible. I wanted to make my brother visible and also to try to understand myself the complexity of his situation, why, even if help is offered, it is often a matter of pride not to accept it.

I write as an able-bodied person and accept fully the ironies implicit in that privilege. And my brother was not further handicapped by poverty or by being unable to speak the language of the health care system. He had the advantages of a disability pension, a good health insurance plan, full mental capacity, and a caring, proactive family. And yet it was not until the final days of his life that the medical establishment and health care professionals seemed to work for him, not against him. How much worse is every single aspect of daily life for those who are disabled, poor, and alone.

Multiple sclerosis is a chimerical, maddening disease. I have only portrayed my brother's struggle with it, and I am responsible for any erroneous statements or assumptions. It should be said that Dave's diagnosis (after a year-long wait for an MRI in British Columbia) and his subsequent interactions with the Ontario medical establishment (emergency rooms, WheelTrans, assisted living and home-care organizations, and the dizzying complexity of cancer treatment regimes) happened during what I can only hope was the nadir of health care efficiency in Canada. And technology too has improved—a small example: turning a tap to wash his hands became almost impossible for my brother. Just before he died, I was about to purchase (for $400, as I recall) one of those brand-new heat-activated faucets, which are now ubiquitous in airports and public buildings. But are they cheap and readily installed in independent-living units?

And then people ask: what would your brother think of this book? As a shy man, he would perhaps have resisted the telling of his story, but he would understand and respect my reasons for telling it. He felt strongly about the rights of the disabled, and he supported unequivocally the impulse to protest and to make clear for the purpose of making better.

For their care, encouragement, and personal or professional support during Dave's final years, after his death, and during the writing of this book, I thank Franklyn Griffiths, Kate West, Ian Burgham, Lorne Rhamey, Susan Cheeseman Joyce, and Judy Sceviour Evans and other kind people in Kirkland Lake (which has revived considerably, I am told, since my visits there); my agent, Jackie Kaiser; Nancy Flight and Rob Sanders of Greystone Books; my daughter, Katherine; my nephews, Quinn and Gideon Hurdle and Jonathan Scarfe; Suki Kaiser; and her mother, Caroline Orr.

But I could not have written this book without the support, good humor, and imaginative engagement of my sister, Sara. Opening the door on family history is a risky enterprise; family members may not agree on the extent to which painful subjects should be confronted. And people have different memories of how things happened. Sara read each draft carefully, sympathetic to my desire to be truthful. She made wonderful suggestions, both practical and creative, and helped me to retrieve forgotten pieces of our growing up. I hope that this book is true to the spirit of our family and that it is seen as a celebration of our brother's life. Clearly we are, still, the three of us.